"It's amazing when you meet a kindred heart, as Jenn and I originally connected around the worship of God and a love for His presence. Now, after many years of friendship, our shared love of family, food, authenticity, community, and the power of gathering around the table are also some of the things I love most about this woman. I know this book will bring a great refreshing to your heart, as you allow Jenn to lead you into *All Things Lovely*."

—DARLENE ZSCHECH

"In *All Things Lovely* Jenn teaches us that what we magnify matters, and what happens when you magnify the Lord is everything else becomes dim. What a beautiful reminder to keep our eyes and thoughts on Jesus alone. I love the way Jenn helps us apply this to every area of our lives—even in keeping our homes organized—because in that we discover the peace that order and health bring. Jenn is the most hospitable and generous hostess and I've been privileged to experience for myself the way she lives what she shares in the words of this book."

—LAURIE CROUCH

"I don't think I've ever met anyone who thrived on creating beauty and excellence as much as Jenn Johnson. She amazes me. And then when you add to that her amazing ability to host people in a way that makes them feel like royalty, you have an unusual gift indeed. Imagine capturing all those qualities and putting them into a book. *All Things Lovely* is just that. A book that inspires beauty, excellence, and love for people. It will inspire the wisdom of creativity in all who read it—even those who feel they don't have a creative bone in their body. I encourage you to immerse yourself into this joyful journey and watch how Jesus increases the impact of your life in ways that delight His heart and strengthen people."

—BILL JOHNSON,
Bethel Church, Redding, CA, author of *Dreaming with God* and *Born for Significance*

"*All Things Lovely* isn't simply the title of this book, it's the theme of Jenn's entire life! Whether leading thousands to worship Jesus in a packed arena or belly laughing around the table with friends in her home, she compels others toward the spirit and substance of loveliness, as well as the relational reality of the belovedness that God alone graces us with. This is a work of art you'll treasure!"

—LISA HARPER

"Jenn is hospitality grace in a bottle. Literally, the gift of generosity drips from her bones. Her ability to connect the grace of hosting with the heart of her perfect Heavenly Father is just stunning. You're going to love peeking into her home and life and be completely inspired to live with open hands and heart in the life God has also prepared for you!"

—SHELLEY GIGLIO

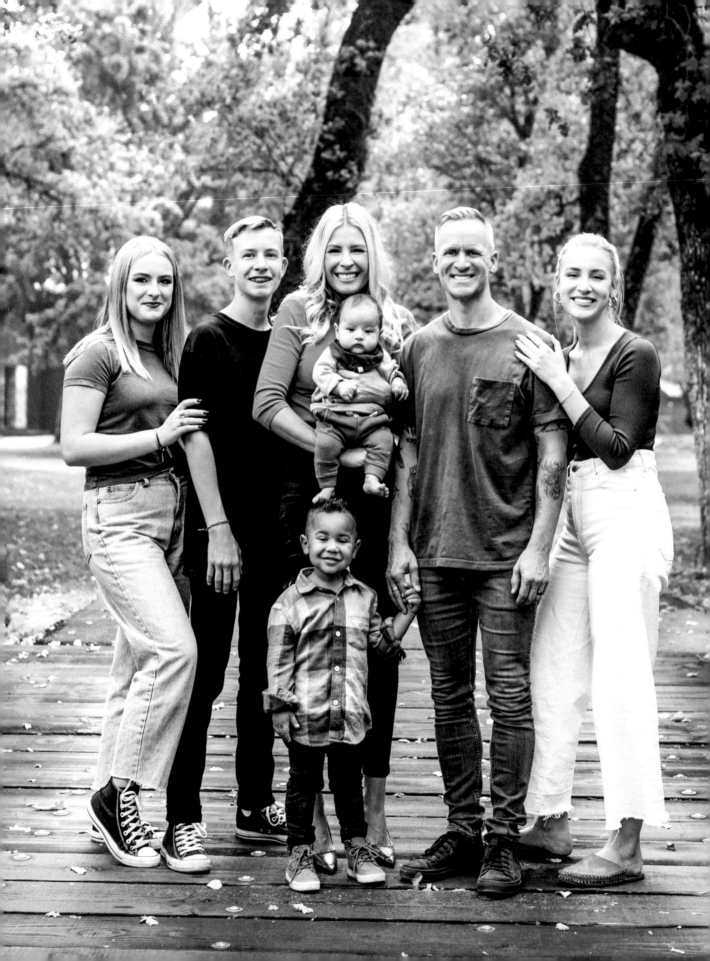

ALL THINGS
LOVELY

Inspiring Health and Wholeness
in Your Home, Heart, & Community

JENN JOHNSON

Photographs by
Heather Armstrong Photography

WORTHY
PUBLISHING

Worthy
Hachette Book Group
1290 Avenue of the Americas, New York, NY 10104
worthypublishing.com
twitter.com/worthypub

First Edition: November 2021

Worthy is a division of Hachette Book Group, Inc.
The Worthy name and logo are trademarks of Hachette Book Group, Inc.

The publisher is not responsible for websites (or their content) that are not owned by the publisher.

The Hachette Speakers Bureau provides a wide range of authors for speaking events. To find out more, go to www.hachettespeakersbureau.com or call (866) 376-6591.

Print book interior design by Shubhani Sarkar, sarkardesignstudio.com

Photographs on pages v (lower left corner), xii, 63, 80–81, 161 are by Caleb Marmolejo.
Photographs on pages 78, 94, 150, 151, 208–209 are by Jordana Griffith.
Photograph on page 157 (bottom) is by @juan,and.angie.
Childhood photos on pages viii, 2, and 96, and the handwritten recipe on 206 are from the author's personal collection.
Photographs on pages 84, 132, and 158 are by Rachel Soh—Bethel Music.
Photographs on pages 86 and 169, bottom, are by Jessica Aitken—Bethel Music.

All other photographs are copyright © 2021 Heather Armstrong Photography.

Library of Congress Cataloging-in-Publication Data
Names: Johnson, Jenn, 1982- author.
Title: All things lovely : inspiring health and wholeness in your home, heart, and community / Jenn Johnson.
Description: First edition. | New York, NY : Worthy, 2021.
Identifiers: LCCN 2021023038 | ISBN 9781546015727 (hardcover) | ISBN 9781546015741 (ebook)
Subjects: LCSH: Christian women—Religious life. | Christian life—Biblical teaching.
Classification: LCC BV4527 .J63545 2021 | DDC 248.8/43—dc23
LC record available at https://lccn.loc.gov/2021023038

ISBNs: 978-1-5460-1572-7 (hardcover); 978-1-5460-1574-1 (ebook)

Printed in Canada

FRI

10 9 8 7 6 5 4 3 2 1

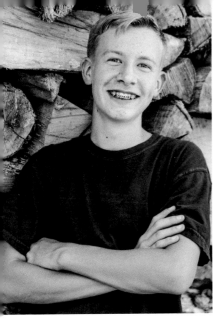

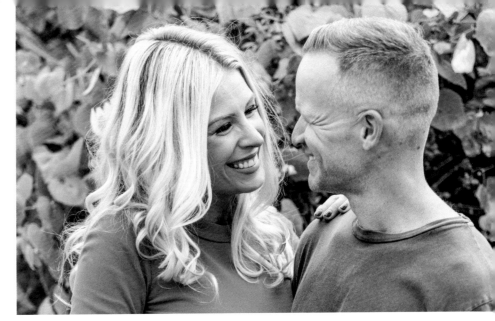

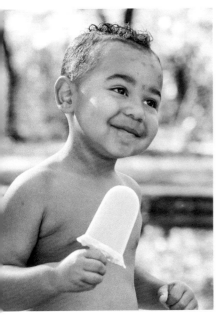

I DEDICATE THIS BOOK

to my love, Brian Johnson,
and our five incredible kids,
Haley Bren, Tèa Kate,
Braden Tyler, Ryder Moses,
and Malachi Judah.
I love you all
more than anything.

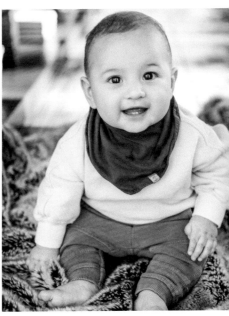

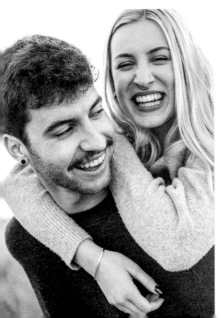

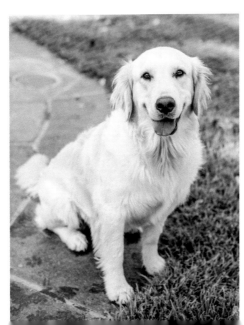

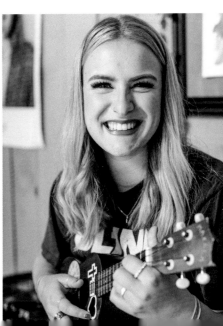

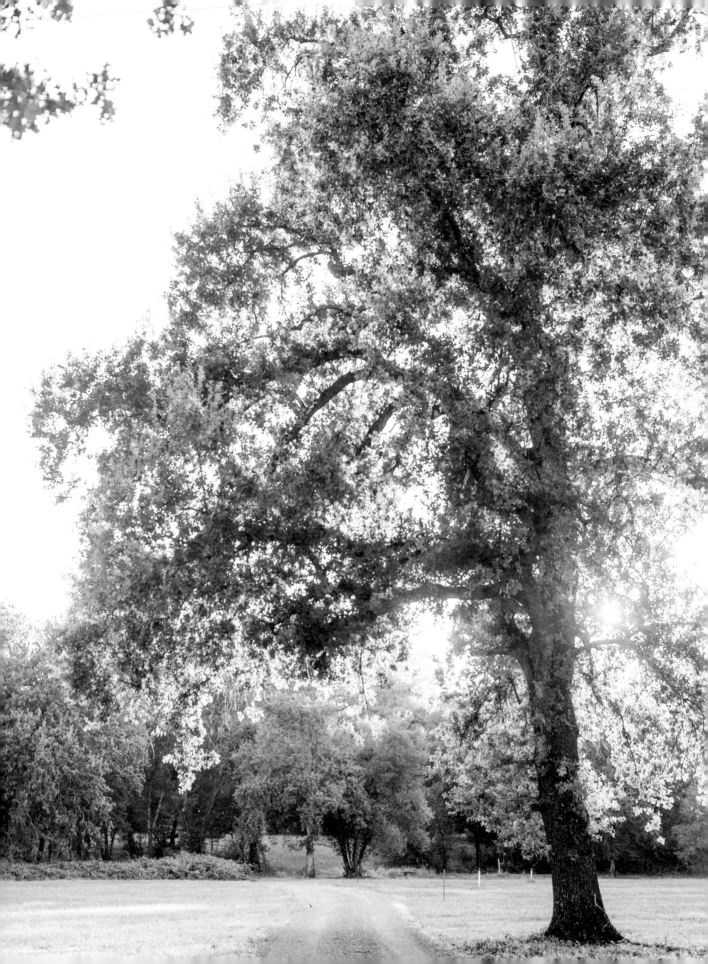

CONTENTS

Introduction.......................ix

Part 01 HOME

Ch. 01   Get Your House in Order 3

Ch. 02   Acknowledge the Mess 13

Ch. 03   Room by Room 21

Part 03 HEALTH

Ch. 08   Feeling Out of Order 91

Ch. 09   The Power of Belief 95

Ch. 10   Your Body 99

Ch. 11   Work, Play, Rest 133

Part 02 HEART

Ch. 04   Lay It All Down 61

Ch. 05   Clarity and Purity 67

Ch. 06   Healing 77

Ch. 07   Worship 85

Part 04 HOSPITALITY

Ch. 12   Community 149

Ch. 13   Gathering 167

Ch. 14   Hosting 181

Conclusion
ALL THINGS LOVELY..... 211

Acknowledgments............. 216

Appendixes

WHAT'S IN MY KITCHEN 220

MEASUREMENT EQUIVALENTS 222

FOOD STORAGE GUIDE 223

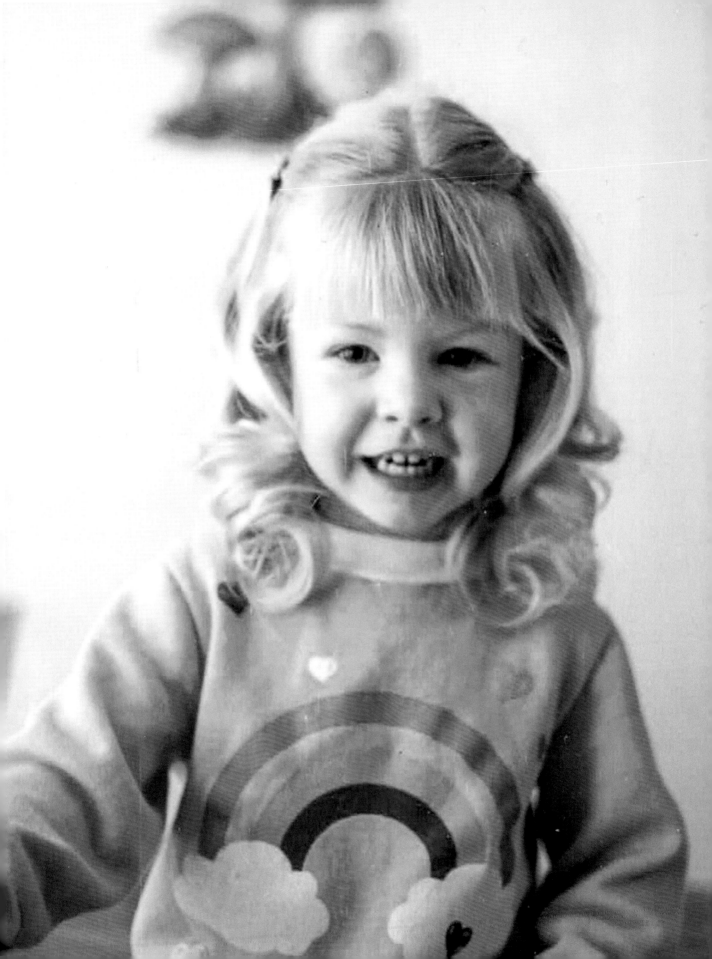

Introduction

My biggest prayer for you as you read this book is that it encourages and strengthens your relationship with God, which in turn will help you reflect and magnify Him in all you say and do.

No matter what your situation in life is right now, I can almost guarantee—like mine—it's a lot to deal with. I wrote this book to inspire you to get healthy emotionally, spiritually, and physically; to deal with everything messy in your life (no junk drawers); and to challenge you to practically love people in the area of hospitality—from opening your home as a host to opening your heart for the possibility of adoption. Welcoming people into your *real* life (the good parts and the ugly parts), being there for them in the highs and lows of life, and loving them like Jesus did, encouraging, teaching, healing, and eating together. One of my favorite things about Jesus is how He met with people in their homes.

This book allows you to "come as you are"— bringing with you all your hopes, your goals, your ideas, and everything messy in your life. I hope to inspire you to create space in your life for all things holy and lovely—in your home, in your heart, in maintaining your health, and in the hospitality you provide as a host.

As for me, my life is an absolute circus most days! I'm married to Brian, my amazing husband of twenty-one years (he is the MAN). We have five incredible kids, ranging from one year old to twenty years old—three are biological and two are adopted. We have a dog, three cats, a few goats and chickens . . . and thankfully they all live outside. And because all of that isn't enough work on its own (don't worry, we have help), I like to grow a few things in my garden on the side and I LOVE to cook. Brian and I have been leading Bethel Music and our local worship team for more than twenty years. We love to worship God and serve the local and global church, singing, writing, teaching, and raising up leaders. And we've been working on renovating and rebuilding our house for the last nine years. (Yes, nine. And that explains why we're crazy. Ha!) Our life is definitely . . . full. Very full. It's a wild ride, but we love it and wouldn't have it any other way.

We love inviting people into our home; I often joke with Brian that we should replace our front door with a revolving door since we have people coming and going all day every day. We love hosting—from birthdays, baby showers, to holidays and everything in between; we take every opportunity to celebrate life. We keep a lot of extra food on hand because our house is known for being open to friends, family, and team members who need to "stop by and talk"; and our kids' friends know they have a place to hang out multiple times a week.

While we love having people over all the time, no matter how hard we try to keep our home and our lives clean and "presentable" . . . it's impossible. But I've learned that inviting people in often means inviting them into your mess. With this book, I want to invite you into our home and our family.

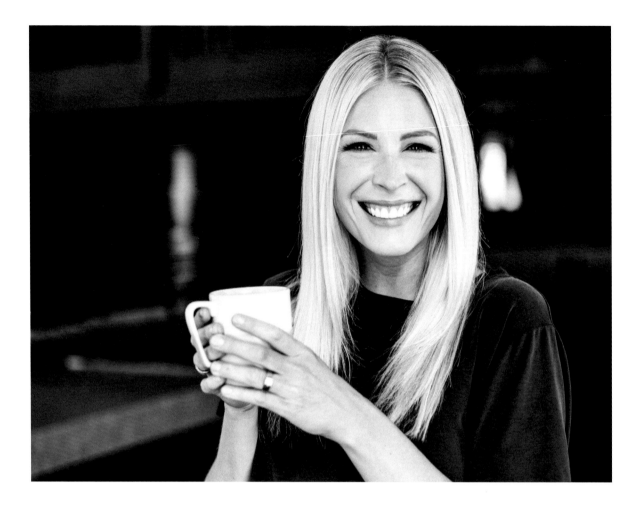

Our real lives. For example, am I currently looking at a huge pile of laundry that needs to be folded as I write this? Yes, yes I am.

Throughout this book, I want to share wisdom, tips, and insights I've learned from cleaning out the emotional, physical, and spiritual junk drawers in my life, finding the peace that order and health allow and the joy and strength community brings. My greatest tip: find what works for you and your family. If the way the contents of my fridge look inspires you, by all means, take notes. But my fridge isn't perfect. It just works for our family. That's all. The same goes for how I take care of my body and how I host people. The point is, I want to be very clear that God (and hopefully this book) will help you find what works for you.

We serve a happy and holy God who wants to lead and guide us in every area of our lives, and this book is a celebration of just that. I pray that as you read this book, it will help you become passionate and intentional in every area of your life, healthy, clutter-free, and that you will love Jesus and people even more.

So, welcome into our lives. I love each and every one of you, and even if I don't know you yet, I can't wait to hang out and eat delicious food in heaven with you and God. The party will be at my house.

xoxo

Jenn

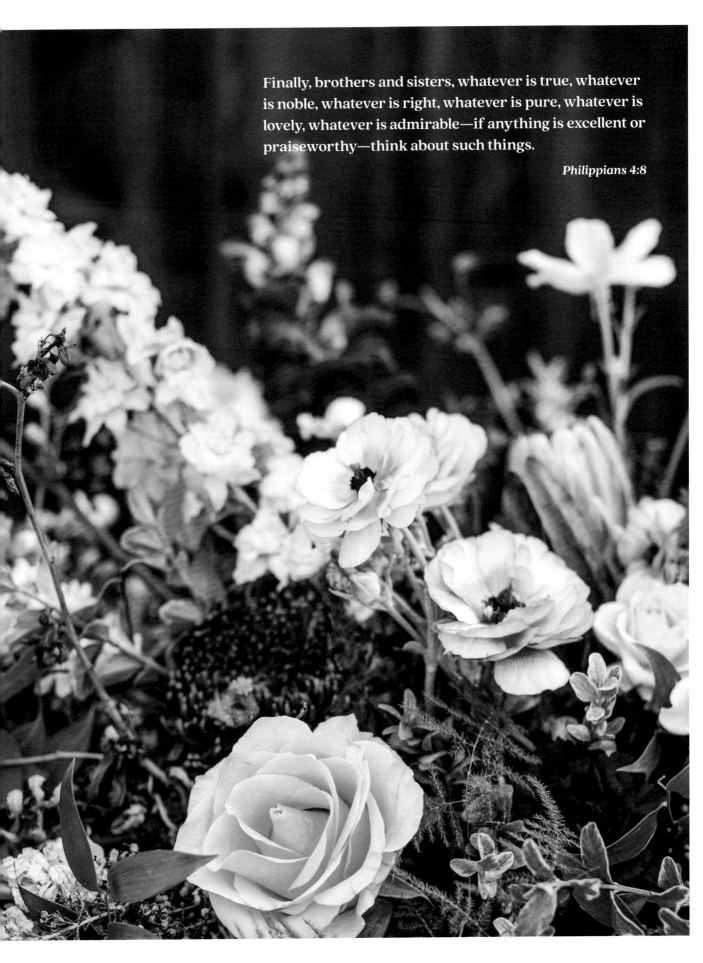

Finally, brothers and sisters, whatever is true, whatever is noble, whatever is right, whatever is pure, whatever is lovely, whatever is admirable—if anything is excellent or praiseworthy—think about such things.

Philippians 4:8

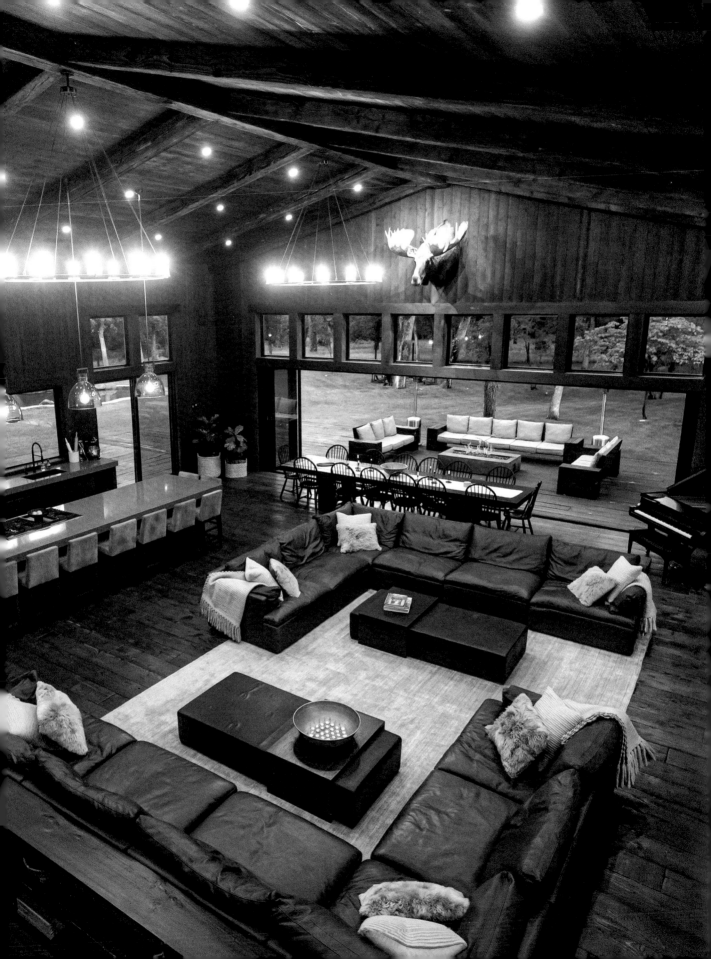

Part 01 | HOME

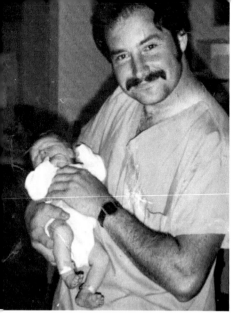
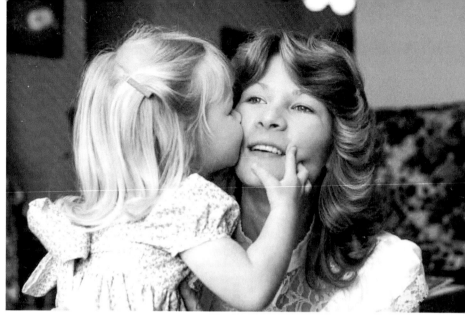
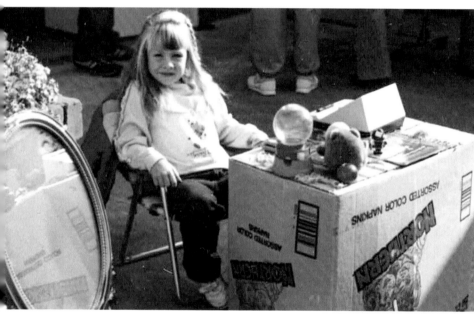
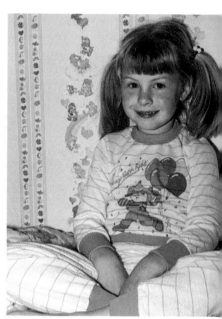
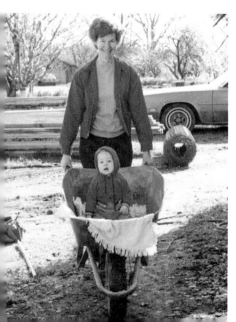
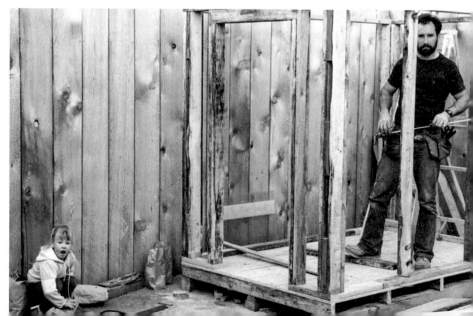

Ch. 01 | GET YOUR HOUSE IN ORDER

I grew up in beautiful Northern California. My parents are amazing and it's clear where my love for God, community, the church, and hard work began.

My parents both worked full-time, my dad a logger and my mom a nurse and hairstylist, and they were both leaders in the church. I spent a lot of time as a kid playing in the redwood forest with my brother, sister, and cousins or at our grandma Jane's house helping her work in her huge garden. She definitely had a green thumb; she grew vegetables, herbs, flowers, and trees. To this day, one of my favorite things is the smell of a tomato plant. My childhood was wonderful—filled with school, Bible study, friends, summer camps, youth events, birthday parties, baby and wedding showers, church twice on Sunday, and a *lot* of potlucks. We had a very happy home. And whether it was my dad waking me up singing a country song, one of our family members playing an instrument, or the newest Christian tune blaring from somewhere . . . there was almost *always* music in our house.

Beginning with when my parents got married, and still to this day, their home has been a "fixer-upper" (they've lived in and remodeled seven houses). Growing up, there was usually some part of our house being remodeled so, clearly, I got my love of that from them. Brian and I are living in our third fixer-upper. I think there's something spiritual about renovation. It is definitely a God concept to restore and make all things new.

My mom let us kids decorate our rooms the way we liked (within good measure), and I loved to decorate and change my room design frequently—from Holly Hobbie to Rainbow Brite to Anne Geddes and sunflowers. I couldn't wait to have my own house one day to decorate. A big house with a big family, maybe a dog and a garden just like my grandma Jane's.

About ten years ago, after three kids, four houses, and two remodels, Brian and I decided that we wanted to find our forever home, which for me meant a house like the one in the movie *Father of the Bride* or *Home Alone*. The place where our kids would grow up and our grandkids would eventually come visit.

We dreamed of a house with a huge great room so we could host people . . . a lot of people. Gatherings and community have always been a big part of our lives, having both grown up in small towns and small churches. At the time, we were a few years into leading the worship team at Bethel, and we were experiencing a lot of growth. When we had the whole team over to our house once a month to worship, pray, eat, and hang out together, we were bursting at the seams; there seemed to be people coming out doors and windows!

We also dreamed of having land, and it felt like this was the time for that as well. Both of us love the outdoors so much. We both grew up near the woods so lots of trees were a must. We wanted the kind of

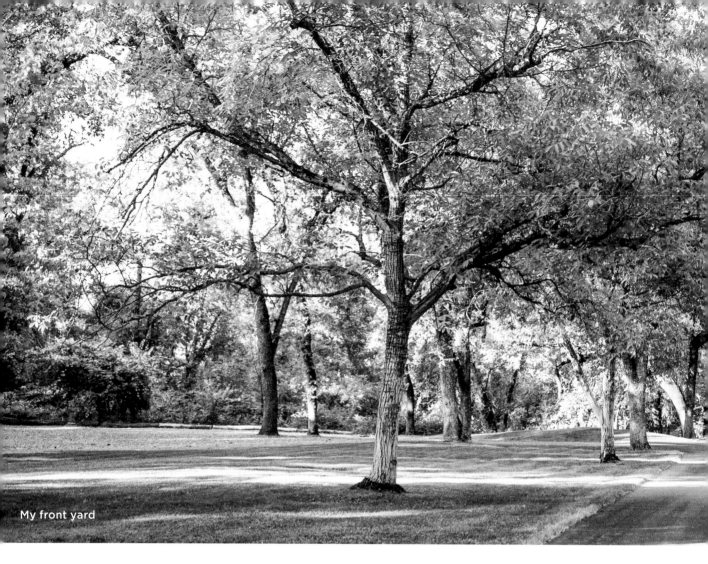

My front yard

land where we could have a garden (lots of tomato plants), animals, a pool, and space for our kids to run around and explore. We dreamed of a property where we could host all kinds of gatherings inside or out, like dinner parties, holidays, retreats, birthdays, baby showers, staff meetings, and album release parties. We wanted to spread out—and we dreamed of a beautiful property where people could come to relax in nature, have fun, get refreshed, be inspired, connect, and feel loved by us and Jesus.

When our two oldest kids were in school, I would take our youngest, Braden (who was three at the time), with me to drive around looking at houses with land. Brian and I were in love with a particular area around Redding—wooded acres, close to town

and the airport, small herds of animals, orchards and gardens everywhere, and, most importantly . . . lots of huge, beautiful trees.

I'll never forget the day I found it—*the* house. Braden had fallen asleep in the car seat and I was driving around our favorite area looking for anything for sale. I found a roughly paved little road, and at the end there was an overgrown property entrance. I couldn't see the house from the road, so I decided to drive in. I figured if it wasn't abandoned, as it looked to be, I would just apologize for the intrusion. As I drove onto the property, the road wound around to an old bridge over a beautiful creek that led up to the house. It was quiet. *It was magical.* Overgrown and abandoned . . . but magical.

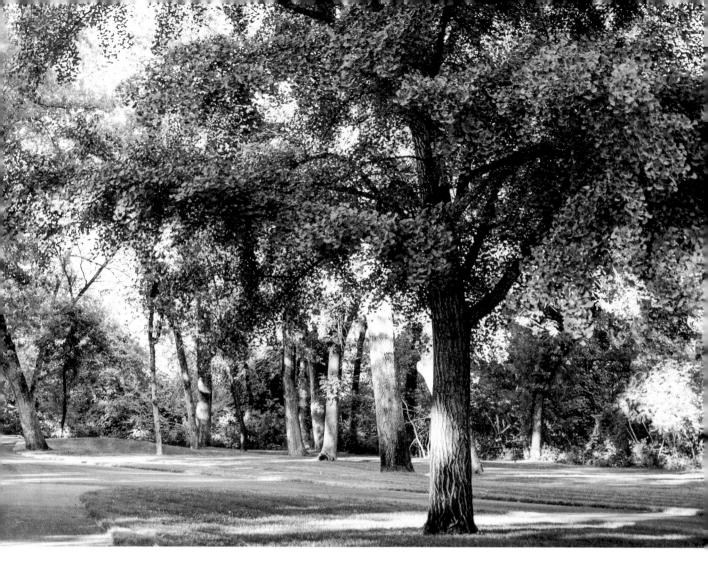

I doubt it would have impressed many people, but I saw what it *could* be! SO much potential. I imagine that's how God looks at our lives sometimes. Never overwhelmed or hopeless . . . He always sees us as full of potential no matter how much work is needed.

The tiny shack of a house definitely fell into the run-down category, and the land itself felt like a jungle (or a secret garden), with an insane number of blackberry bushes and overgrown *everything*. But it was beautiful and I knew it could be the perfect home even though it was in shambles. I grabbed my phone to call Brian and told him to come see it. When he drove up, he smiled, his eyes filled with excitement. I remember it like it was yesterday; we walked around the property imagining how we could clean it up, where a garden could go, and what we would change. It was perfect.

We called our realtor and he made a few calls and found out the property was owned by the next-door neighbor. It was on twenty acres, it hadn't been updated since the 1970s, and no one had lived in it for years. There was only one problem . . . it wasn't for sale. But we had a vision, so we figured why not ask if the neighbor would be willing to sell? Our realtor contacted him and (miracle!) he *was* willing to sell! We were over-the-moon excited. After a few days we started escrow, hoping it would be quick . . . but it wasn't. The crazy back-and-forth lasted forever. As we encountered and overcame one hurdle after another, months went by (the owner lost the deed and a million other crazy things), and we wondered if our dream would ever happen.

In the midst of all this, we were going through a lot of challenges at church as well. A few key people on our worship team were moving and it really affected what we had worked so hard to build; plus, there were some other difficult dynamics and "growing pains" we were having to work out. Brian and I were arguing a lot from the stress of dealing with it all emotionally.

At some point during this trying season, Brian and I flew to England to lead worship for an event, and it was nice to be away from the house escrow drama as well as the drama that was happening with our team. The trip came as a welcomed break, especially because the kids were staying home with Grandma on this trip (hallelujah!), so even the long flight felt like a vacation.

One night while we were there, a woman I didn't know came up to me during prayer ministry time at the end of the service and asked if she could pray for me. I love receiving prayer; I'll let just about anyone pray for me (unless I get a weird feeling), and this lady had a very peaceful presence and actually reminded me of a close friend. So I said, "Of course."

For the next two hours, she led me through an incredible inner healing session. She told me to ask God, "What lies have I been believing?" Instantly, this is what I heard God say: *You believe that you haven't loved well, and you haven't led well. Because if you had, no one would leave you.* I started sobbing. That was the lie, loud and clear. And I could feel it being uprooted like a weed. Just like in gardening when things grow, as the church and our team had, weeds had grown too. They needed to be pulled out and this lie was one of them. I told her what God had shown me and she said, "Thank You, Father, for showing her the lie. Now I ask You to show her a picture of the truth." Instantly God showed me a scene from the prodigal son story in the Bible—and it was like watching a movie and fast-forwarding to the

exact part I needed to see . . . the part when the son is leaving his home, his family, and his father. I felt God say to me, *The father didn't chase after his son in the story. He let him go. Sometimes, even in family, to love them well means you have to . . . let them go.*

Let. Them. Go. That was it. That's what I had to do.

One by one, faces came to mind—people who wanted to leave "home," and whom I needed to let go. I repented right there for wanting them to stay and trying to control them because I thought I knew what was best for them. But it had become clear that it wasn't my decision to make. I needed to not only have an open hand to welcome anyone who came onto the team, but also to accept the decision of anyone who left.

She prayed with me through a few more things she was hearing from God and gave me a huge hug. The room that had once been packed with thousands of people now had only a couple left, who were waiting on us to turn out the lights. The woman, who told me her name was Helena, handed me her phone number and told me I could call her anytime if I needed anything. I thanked her again and again, my shirt soaked with tears, but my heart ten pounds lighter.

I told Brian about my healing encounter with God (and Helena), and he was so happy for me. It also made him realize he needed, and wanted, the same thing for himself. We headed home to California the next day, and Brian ended up having a phone conversation with Helena a few days later. Here's where it gets even more fun: this woman knew nothing about our dream-house-shack-land situation, yet, as she was praying with Brian, God showed her an image of a house that had been abandoned and overgrown with "briars," also called . . . blackberry bushes. Brian was wide-eyed as Helena described what she saw: "I see this house as a picture of your heart. God wants to untangle and remove the thorns, restore it, and enlarge it." What?! Amazing! And God's timing for this could not have been more perfect.

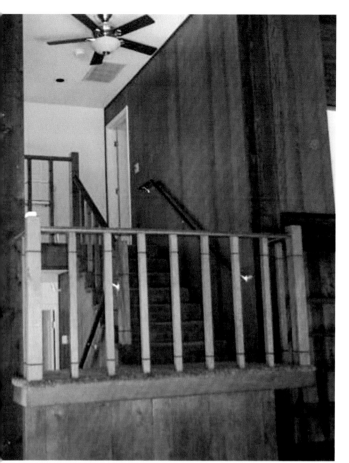

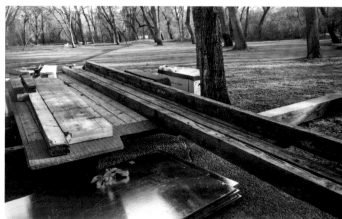

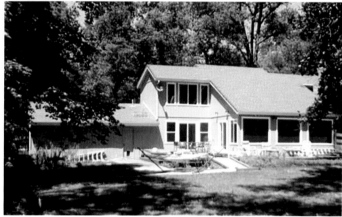

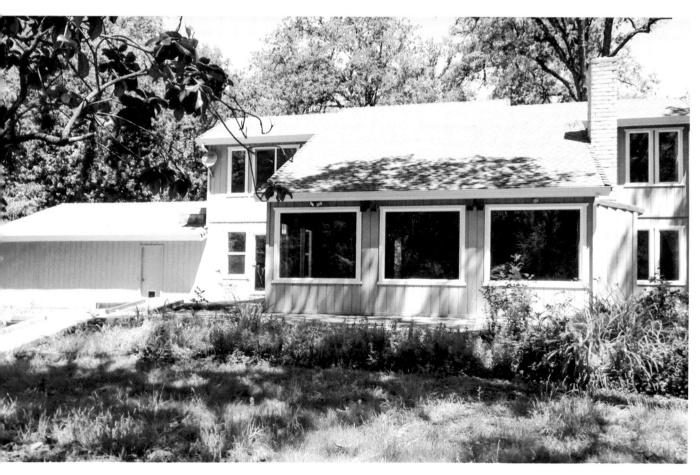

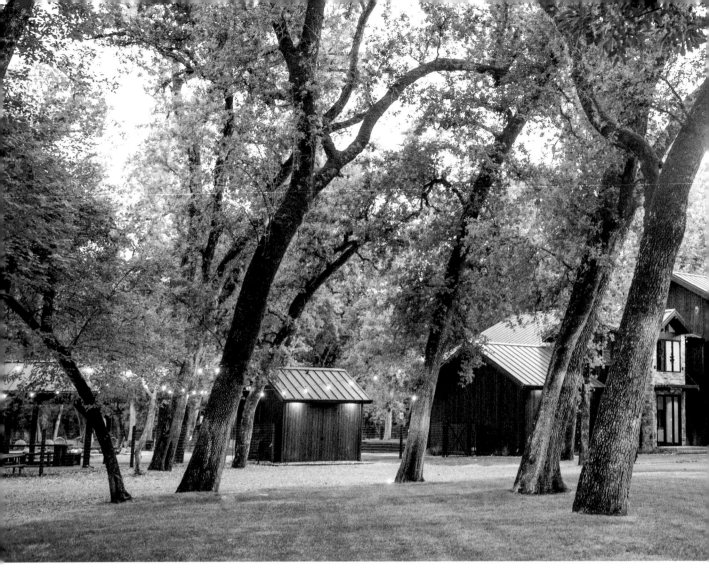

Our hearts being healed and restored and the restoration of this house and property were connected! Of course. It made so much sense. It's just like God to parallel something in the natural and the spiritual.

Shortly after we had this revelation, our realtor called. After ten long months, our house escrow closed! We knew the timing wasn't a coincidence. Driving to our house that day, I heard God say to me, *I didn't want to give you your promise until your hearts were ready for it*. He wasn't holding out on us; He just wanted our hearts to be free and ready for what He had in store for us. Like when you pull all the weeds out of a garden bed before you plant something.

Over the last nine years, we have worked extra hard to turn that shack on the overgrown land into a dream home on gorgeous property. We just kept dreaming and hosting and dreaming again, going waaaaay beyond the dream we first envisioned when we found the house. It hasn't been easy, though; the journey has taken a lot of blood, sweat, and tears. (Especially with our being clean freaks and living in a state of constant construction for nine years.) We've gone through low lows, heartache, and hardships. But God's been with us through it all.

Our house has become everything we could have ever dreamed of and more. It's been an incredible

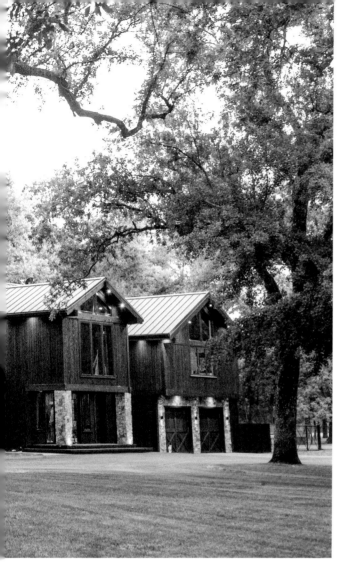

feel . . . "at home" . . . part of a community. And that is exactly what we dreamed it could be.

In Isaiah 38:1 the prophet tells another one of God's servants, Hezekiah, to "put your house in order." It's one of those phrases in the Bible that feels like it's in bold print for me. Although it's written as a warning from Isaiah to Hezekiah that he's going to die (yikes), the point is that he's telling him to get everything in order and take care of things in his life that need attention. God actually wanted to show mercy to Hezekiah; after Hezekiah heard this prophecy, he prayed to God and God added fifteen years to his life (Isa. 38:5). Perhaps an application of this get-your-house-in-order verse is that when God is doing something life-changing, He tells us to prepare for it, to leave nothing buried, hidden, or avoided. No unhandled business. *No junk drawers.* I love the charge of "Put your house in order"—and I believe "house" refers to our *whole* lives: our homes, our physical health, our spiritual hearts, and our connection to community, four things that are often interwoven.

I know many of you holding this book right now feel the chaos of life—whether you're a parent of little ones, a grandparent, or single with one room to call your own. We all need simplicity, order, and a space that makes us happy and peaceful. I believe we all want to be able to open up a closet—or start a conversation or begin a new relationship—and not feel chaotic when we see the clutter we haven't dealt with.

I hear you.

This book will help you empty the junk drawers. *All the junk drawers.* Everyone has them somewhere (in our homes, hearts, and bodies). It's nothing to be ashamed of, just something to be honest about, because then it becomes one hundred percent possible to get those drawers into beautiful order. If you put the work in, you can and will get to a place that feels clear, clean, and peaceful. You can and will breathe easy and know there is nothing hidden or ignored.

You need courage, though—no doubt about that. Whether it's old hurts, old parking tickets,

space for us, our kids, our friends, and the million other people God has brought to walk through our doors and to sit around our table. Though it was a long process from beginning to end, we were intentional with every decision we made, wanting it to be a space curated with love, beauty, and excellence. We host worship sessions, retreats, singles mixers, Bible studies, youth group events, and countless parties of every type. There's always lots of good food in the kitchen for whoever comes by. Our house is known as a refuge for kids who need a safe place; it's a space where people can come to get advice and prayer. Where they can have fun, connect, worship, feel known, feel loved, maybe pet a goat, and ultimately

Get Your House in Order

or old habits, there's usually something shoved back somewhere in the dark corners of our lives and we need courage to bring it to the light. What I've learned is that clutter will only (and always) breed more clutter and chaos. No sense in hiding it, ignoring it, or pretending it's not affecting you. No, we are going to face all of our junk drawers together. We're going to pull everything out, go through it, and get our whole lives into shape.

These transformations often start emotionally and spiritually and then you see the results physically. It's the same for your home, health, and heart. "Put your house in order" means having a holistic vision for all parts of your life. For example, if you read the Bible and pray all the time, but you eat junk and don't exercise . . . you're not "healthy" holistically. When you choose to live holistically healthy, you'll know what you have and where it is (every mismatched sock will finally meet its mate), your heart will be free, your body will be full of energy, and your house will be in order. You'll probably want to have people over and throw a great party. (I'll give you recipes and more to help you with that too!)

No more sweeping things under the rug. It's time to deal with it.

We all have junk drawers—whatever those might hold—but I also recognize we're not all in the same place. Some of us need emotional purging ASAP. Some of us are feeling crushed under the weight of bitterness or stuck in a rut of unhealthy eating or exhaustion. Some of us need to literally dig into our closetful of clothes and give away about half of them. Some of us need to have those difficult conversations we've been avoiding. (And don't feel bad if it's all of the above! You've got this.) We all need renovation or a good purge somewhere, if not in multiple areas of our lives.

But don't be overwhelmed! Let the Holy Spirit guide you. And this book will help!

When you start taking on those junk drawers and getting your house in order, you will see many fruits of the Spirit in your life.

So . . . are you ready to tackle some junk?

Pause and consider:

1 | **Start by inviting the Holy Spirit** into this process with you, even if you're new to experiencing God's Holy Spirit or have never done something like this. Listen for any internal promptings, instincts, pictures, or words.

2 | **Take note.** Whether it's on paper, in your journal, or on your phone, write down anything you get from the Holy Spirit—even if it seems like a stretch, a challenge, or involves an unexpected area of your life. *A verse, a person, a drawer in your house, anything. Even if it's something random, like an apple, and doesn't make sense . . . ask Him to tell you more about it. He will. And you can always ask God questions! Like, "Who do I need to forgive?"; "Who do I need to help?"; or "Where do I start in putting my house in order?"* God is always speaking and wants to talk to you about every detail of your life. The good and the parts that need work. He is a kind and loving Father.

3 | **Display your word from God.** One of my favorite Scriptures is at the end of this chapter. Whatever God speaks to you or whatever Scripture He's highlighting for you, put it in a place where you'll see it often—like your home screen, your bathroom mirror, in the kitchen, next to your front door, or in your car.

Staying connected to what God is speaking to you is important. I love church and how God speaks through leaders, but it's also important to stay in His Word daily and listen for His voice and what He's speaking directly to you.

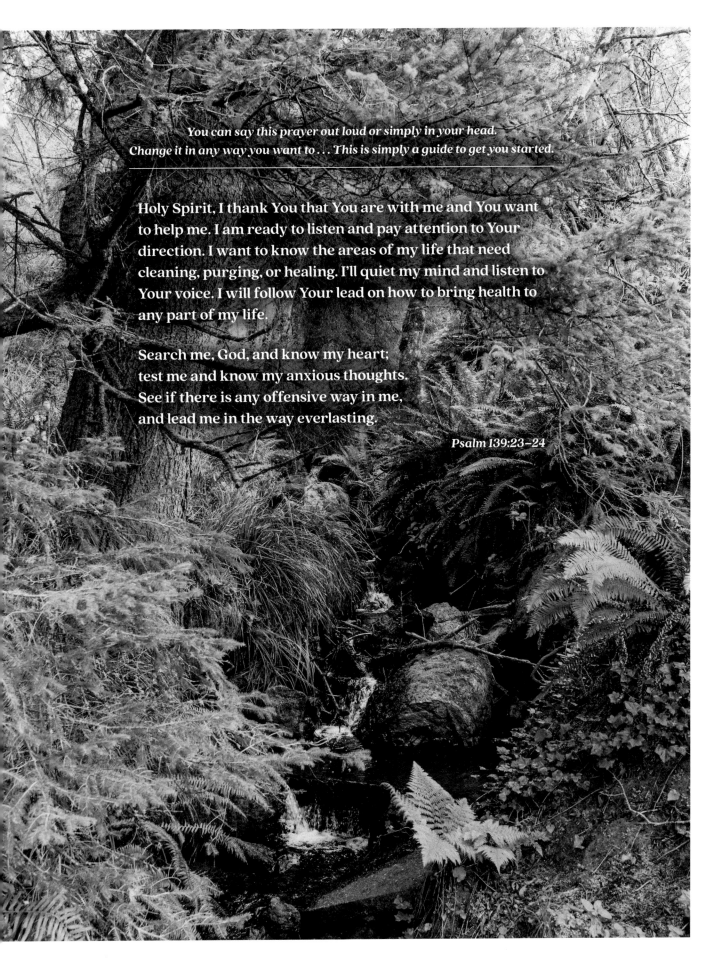

You can say this prayer out loud or simply in your head.
Change it in any way you want to . . . This is simply a guide to get you started.

Holy Spirit, I thank You that You are with me and You want to help me. I am ready to listen and pay attention to Your direction. I want to know the areas of my life that need cleaning, purging, or healing. I'll quiet my mind and listen to Your voice. I will follow Your lead on how to bring health to any part of my life.

Search me, God, and know my heart;
test me and know my anxious thoughts.
See if there is any offensive way in me,
and lead me in the way everlasting.

Psalm 139:23–24

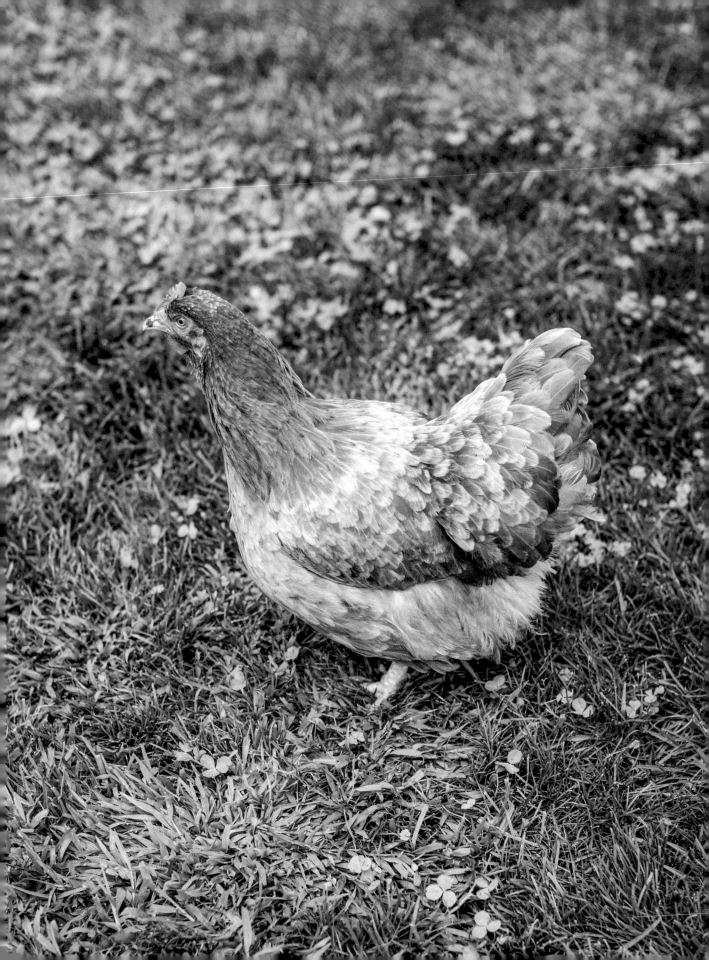

Ch. 02 | ACKNOWLEDGE THE MESS

You know those moments when you lose yourself in something—a movie, a sport, a book, music, or another activity—and time disappears and the world fades away; you emerge from this state only to realize that five hours have passed and you haven't eaten?

I really lose track of time in a few of the things that I regularly do. The first thing is worship. Whether I am writing a new song alone in my living room or on a stage in front of thousands of people, I completely get "in the zone," consumed with God's presence, and sometimes I totally lose track of time.

Another "zone" I get lost in is hosting. When I throw a party, I buzz around making sure needs are met; things are "zhuzhed" (definition: to make something more interesting or attractive by changing it slightly or adding to it); and cups are full. I'll forget to eat for hours and that is very unlike me! I love good party food.

And another thing I lose track of time doing is . . . organizing. I try to approach everything in life with a "heart of worship"; like Colossians 3:23 says: "Whatever you do, work at it with all your heart, as working for the Lord."

In some things that I do, I have to try hard to have that mind-set—but organizing is not one of those things. I love organizing and the peace it brings. My love of organizing and order began in childhood but has developed a lot over the years. I love helping other people organize their spaces too. Like Marie Kondo says, "I love mess" (and even more when it's someone else's).

I remember when one of my friends was at her wit's end raising two little kids and she'd just had another baby. I called to check on her and she started sobbing; her husband was at work, her house was a mess, and she was at her max stress level. I knew what was needed: containers! Actually, containers were just the start of the help she needed, and I knew it because I'd been there. "Can I help?" I asked. She responded, "Please." I told her I would be on my way over, right after I picked up a few things. When I got to her house, she was so happy and so was I—because as much as I love being a wife/mom/worshipper, et cetera, I equally live for loving and helping people, hosting, and bringing order.

We headed to her kitchen, and both of us started laughing at the chaos surrounding us . . . kids' stuff everywhere, dirty dishes piled high in the sink, a baby on her hip and a little one at her feet . . . she teared up again as she laughed. I understood exactly how she was feeling because I had been there many times. My friend knew she needed help and she was ready to accept it. Her vulnerability in letting me into her messy house was courageous . . . and because of her vulnerability and courage, she got

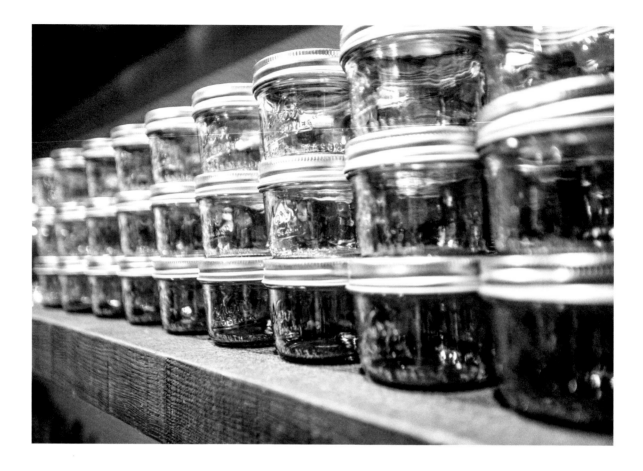

the help she needed. Sometimes, to get the help you need, you have to be humble and ask for it.

So in my friend's house that day, I started by making us some coffee. I poured her a cup and took her baby into my arms, and she set up a movie and snacks for her older kids in the living room. I handed the baby back to her and rolled up my sleeves. We were going to start by tackling the kitchen. First, I loaded the dishes, cleaned the countertops, and prepped her kitchen to make space for some massive upheaval. I smiled and said, "Okay. Everything's gonna come out. Don't panic. It gets worse before it gets better." And it's true . . . sometimes it does get worse before it gets better. Whether it's physical or emotional junk, this is how it seems to go. But believe me, it's worth experiencing the worst to get to the better.

The kitchen makeover took about five hours. I created three piles: trash, errands, and donations. In no time, I had a big pile of trash (lids that didn't fit anything, broken items, processed foods that she didn't want her family eating); a pile of "errands" (library books, friends' containers from dropped-off meals, Target returns); and, last, a large pile of donations (like the fondue set she never used and things from her wedding that she was keeping only because she felt bad about getting rid of them). "Don't keep things in your house that you don't love and use," I coached her. "If you want to keep it because it's a keepsake, then keep it contained in the garage. Not inside your house. That space is limited and precious."

"Sometimes it does get worse before it gets better."

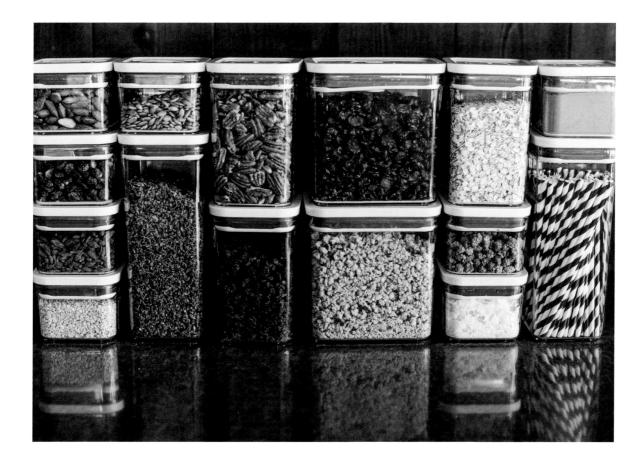

By the fifth hour, we had that kitchen dialed. Every square inch was purged and organized. Airtight containers and mason jars were filled with cereal, baking ingredients, and snacks. (Mason jars are a great, cheap, chic way to organize.) Spices were alphabetized, toddler plasticware was within a toddler's reach; glasses and dishware were safely out of a toddler's reach. The pantry was emptied of everything unwanted or expired and rearranged so that her whole family could see everything they needed to see. Now the kids could be more self-sufficient, often helping themselves, so that she didn't have to run "kitchen command" all the time.

But in the midst of all this sorting and purging, something else changed when I started asking her questions about her life. As I was cleaning cabinets, she began letting out some raw frustrations about how overwhelmed she felt. I listened and gave her any wisdom I was getting from God as she talked. After a little while of emotional pouring-out, I guided the conversation in another direction and asked her to tell me what was amazing in her life right now. Her eyes lit up as she began telling me all the good things. And her frustration turned to gratefulness. It was lovely. No, all of her problems didn't go away, but focusing on gratefulness is a great foundation to work on things that need change. For example, sometimes the baby you prayed for equals 400,000 dirty diapers. A lot of the things she was frustrated about were things she prayed for. Been there.

She went from gratitude to hope. We talked about guarding our words and how they have so much power. I told her that instead of the common go-to expression "My life is so crazy!" (a self-fulfilling prophecy), I would say, "Yes, life is full, but

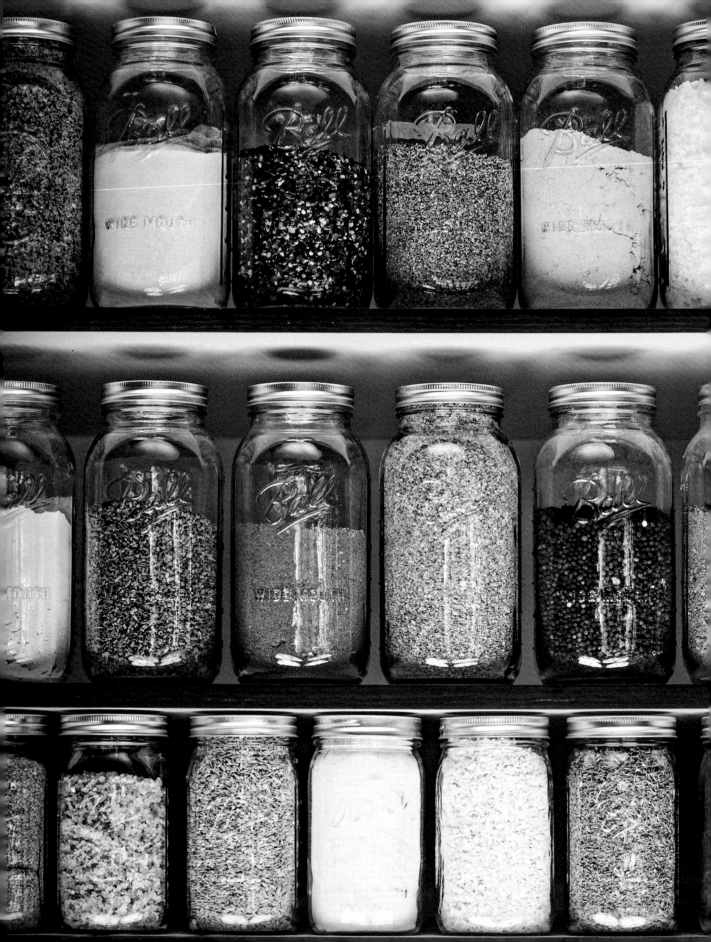

I like it full . . . I just need the Holy Spirit to guide me in prioritizing, organizing, and tackling it all." I reminded her what a good friend she's been to me and others. I told her she's an amazing wife and mom. And now, with an organized kitchen and a grateful heart, life was going to be a little bit easier for her. She welcomed help. The emotional and physical clutter had been acknowledged, sorted out, and dealt with; order was created and hope was restored.

As I left her house that day, her eyes filled with tears again as she thanked me and gave me a huge hug. Life can feel like you're in quicksand sometimes, but that's why Jesus gave us community. That day in her kitchen, my friend received help because of her vulnerability and willingness to receive help! So, acknowledge your needs, acknowledge your mess, and invite someone in. Remember, there are people who love to help! Don't try to do it all yourself. You need help. We all do.

Not everything you face will be complex and intense—sometimes a messy closet is just a messy closet. But remember that the mess in your home might be an indication of some deep and unresolved frustrations in your heart. Therefore, as you start tackling your messy areas, if you hit a wall, you'll know the resistance *could* be coming from something else that's chaotic underneath.

I always go into organization mode with a beautiful image in my mind as the end goal. The image could be the cleaned cabinet itself, or imagining how happy I'll feel when I'm finished. Instead of scrambling the next morning to get our family out the door, I picture us efficiently getting ready and no one becoming upset because they can't find their coat or backpack. (One can dream!) That's the kind of hope that motivates me through a project, big or small. I visualize the end goal. The fruit. And that's a big reason why this book is loaded with photography—to inspire ideas for you too. I want to visually show you a *real* family of seven and their stuff, in their house . . . and how they make it work.

Before we get into the details and go from room to room to help you get your house in order, I want to talk through two principles that have been super helpful to me as I organize my house—or when I help friends: **generosity and stewardship**.

1| **GENEROSITY:** This will have huge practical implications as you organize your home.

Keep only what you love, need, and use. (I would make that sentence light up and *blink* in this book if I could!) If you don't need something in this season, someone else needs it. And if you need it again in the future, trust God—He will provide it again.

Not only does generosity mean you'll be serving and helping others, it also brings you more peace because you aren't drowning in extra stuff you don't need. Let the Holy Spirit speak to you about what you have and be openhanded with everything. Luke 6:38 says, "Give, and it will be given to you. Good measure, pressed down, shaken together, running over, will be put into your lap" (ESV). You don't have to give everything away; you can always sell things online or host a good old-fashioned garage sale. Even then, you can be helping others by putting something they need into their hands at a great price.

2| **STEWARDSHIP:** I've been a thrifty person all my life (thank you, Mom). I love a good deal, discounts, buying in bulk, working the system, and finding the best price for everything I buy. We've had many times in our lives when we could barely pay our bills; and the personal debt we carried from making an album (before we started Bethel Music) was a lot. Even though we have more now, we're just as thrifty. We do our best to take care of what we have and be resourceful. This not only affects how we shop, but also how we constantly declutter and purge our house and property. When you have less to deal with because you purge frequently, it's way easier to maintain order and be a good steward of what you own.

As you go through your house room by room, putting in the effort right now, both the short- and long-term rewards will be worth it. Putting your house in order will not only help everything in your life go more smoothly; an orderly house will help you make the most of your time, and even save you a lot of money. Instead of buying extras simply because you can't find what you have, you will know what's in your house and what you actually need. Instead of fumbling through a messy closet, anyone in the family can find exactly what they need and soon know if it fits or works. Put in the time now, and you'll save time and stress later.

Physical order creates emotional freedom. Even if you can't fully anticipate how amazing it is to be organized, you'll be surprised along the way by how it makes your life better.

pro TIP Buy quality items. When Brian and I first got married, our other newlywed friends were buying a bunch of low-quality, inexpensive furniture. We knew that furniture would get ruined and fall apart quickly, so we waited and saved money until we could afford good-quality items, one at a time. It saved us from having to make repeat purchases as things fell apart, which of course saved us money and time in the long run. All this to say, I never have accumulation as a goal, but rather intentional selection and good stewardship. As you're organizing room by room in your house, be selective. Don't buy it because it "works right now." Think bigger and with longevity in mind.

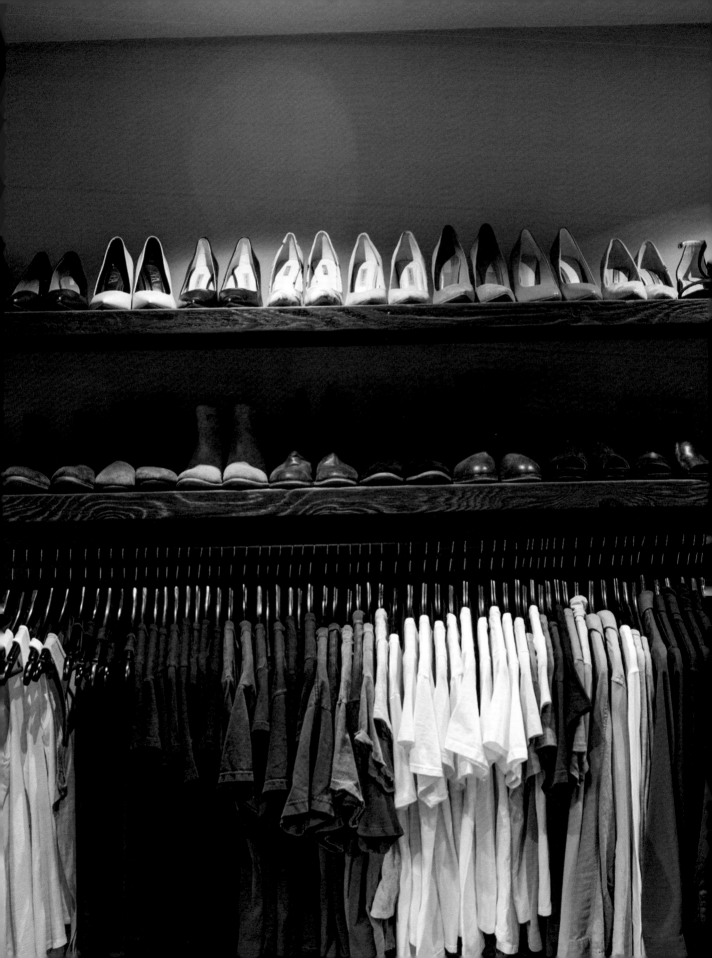

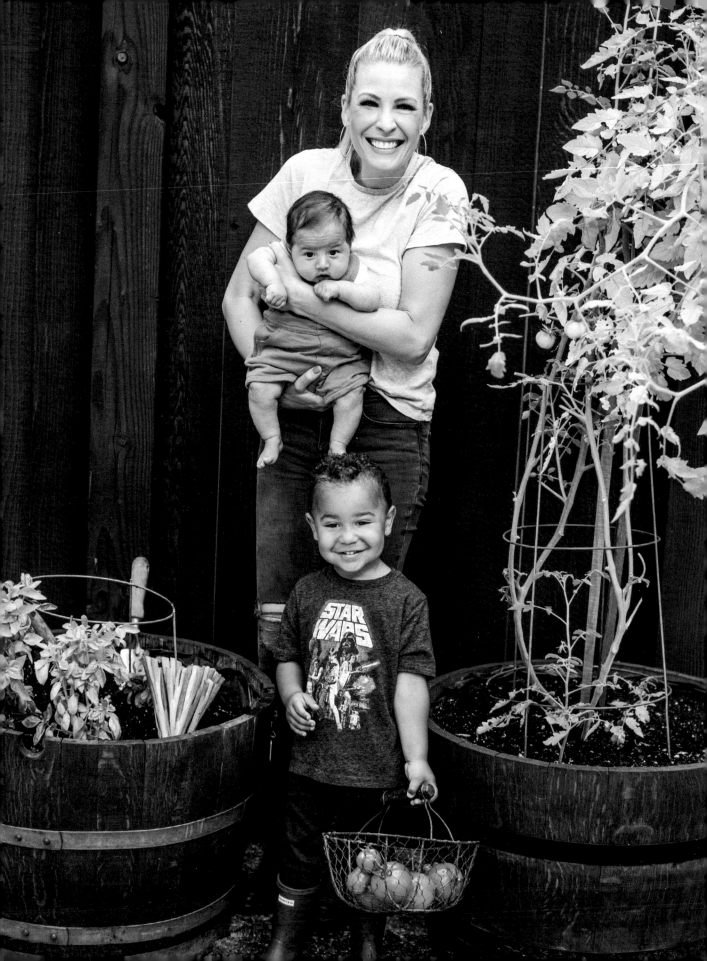

Ch. 03 | ROOM BY ROOM

I love big visions, but I am a detail-oriented person. If I think about organizing my whole house, I get overwhelmed. I like to break up goals into smaller, practical tasks and go one room at a time.

By going through every room in your house and getting rid of the junk, you'll not only have more space in your home, but you'll also have more space emotionally. When our homes are cluttered, often our minds and hearts are too. Go room by room, take it one day, one task, one drawer at a time. Following are some practical tips.

I prepare for house organizing projects by doing three things: I make sure everyone in the house is on the same page with purging and organizing (spouse, kids, roommates); I set up a babysitter and ask a friend or two to help; and I gather a bunch of empty containers.

1. GET EVERYONE ON THE SAME PAGE.

If you're like me, getting everyone in your house on the same page is challenging (especially with a family that includes kids from college age to newborn, like us)—but totally worth it! I learned early on that this house-in-order thing couldn't rest only on my shoulders. I need everyone to be part of the team and agree to some core values. Once that's set up, it's a much easier system to maintain.

For our family, getting everyone on the same page means a daily commitment to order and excellence, not just once a month, or a once-a-year overhaul. When the day ends, we try to put our house back in order so we're ready to start the next day. Specifically, this looks like a "clean up after yourselves" for all the common spaces—like kitchen, bathroom, and main living spaces. I'm more lenient with bedrooms during the week, but dirty laundry piling up in baskets? Nope. Once you're old enough to pour in the detergent, that job is yours.

But let me explain what's behind these rules: **responsibility, self-awareness, and self-esteem**. As a family, we want to take care of what we've been given. We want to be self-aware so that we recognize how we affect our environments and the people around us. When you carry this level of responsibility and awareness, you create stronger self-esteem because you know that you're doing *estimable* things and caring for others. For our kids, this looks like them doing their laundry, taking out the trash, doing dishes, helping to cook, helping to gather firewood, packing their own lunches for school, setting the table, taking care of their animals, and properly cleaning up after their guests leave.

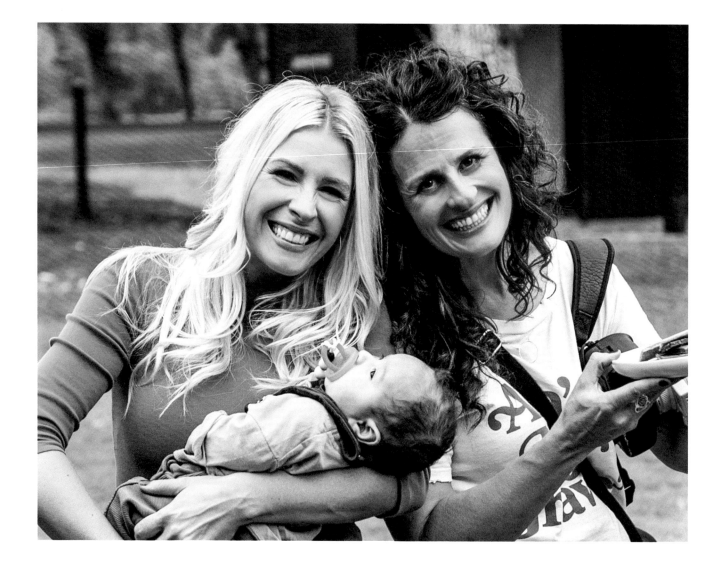

If you live on your own, here's a tip: get your life organized now so that it's easier to keep it that way. Even if you feel like the mess doesn't matter because it's just you dealing with it, I would challenge you to reconsider and think bigger. Order is not just about what level of mess you can tolerate; it's about being a good steward of your space, time, belongings (like keeping your car clean so someone who unexpectedly needs a ride doesn't need a hazmat suit), and money—honoring God with how you take care of all you've been given. One day, you'll probably add a roommate, a spouse, or kids. The good habits you form now will continue to make things easier for you in your next phase in life.

2. GET A BABYSITTER AND ASK A FRIEND OR TWO OVER TO HELP.

Cleaning and organizing while you have little kids at home can feel like brushing your teeth while eating Oreos. If you have little ones, get someone to look after them so you can totally focus on the project you're tackling. Don't invite your kids into the purging process; they'll want to keep things that need to be tossed, like the craft they made out of ice-pop sticks that has only one stick left on it, or your daughter's favorite sequined shirt bearing only one sequin.

Invite a friend over or have your spouse

help. This will also give you motivation and accountability. Maybe get a friend who also wants to organize their home and work on each other's houses! Community has so many beautiful benefits, and helping each other out is one of them. **Life is full and you can't do it all!** The key is asking for help and combining forces. Otherwise, it takes forever to get things done or you never do them.

3. GATHER CONTAINERS.

Although the dream might be having perfectly matching containers (I feel you), don't stress on that part at first. Just get things to the place where they are organized, purged, and contained, especially if you don't want to spend money right now. You can always go back and get the aesthetically pleasing containers later on.

Instead, get together as many baskets or containers as you can find—of various sizes—so that when you pull things out, you have a place to *put* them. The need seems obvious, but I know of many times when someone just dumped everything out and ended up piling most of it right back where it was, because there wasn't anything to contain the order they had created.

In addition to your containers, you're more than likely going to have three other piles when organizing:

1| Trash

2| Give away

3| Errands

You'll need a few grocery bags or boxes. You'll probably find things that need to be fixed or taken somewhere else, so have an "errands" box. (I keep the errands box open, so I'm not tempted to throw it on a shelf and forget about it, and I put each errand's items in their own bag. That way it's simple: grab the bag and drop it at the dry cleaners, or grab the Target return, or grab the friend's stuff I'm returning.) You might also want to ask someone to help you with the errands. There are teenagers everywhere looking for somewhere to drive—pay them to run your errands, or they may be so happy to drive, they might pay you! Ha!

I also use large plastic containers for things I want to keep but that don't require prime real estate in my house. So even if it's not a giveaway or trash, it might be a keepsake or one of those things that get used only a few times a year. It's better for those things to get pulled out of the garage or storage when you need them instead of cluttering the coveted space inside your house.

Ready to get started? You can read straight through now or flip to the area of your house that you're organizing. Having a hard time figuring out where to start? I recommend starting with your favorite place (for me, that's the kitchen). Grab your favorite drink, turn on some music, have a couple of friends over, and get to work.

 Don't start a project that you won't have time to finish, or it will drive you nuts. Allow more time than you think you'll need. If you have a babysitter for two hours, don't expect to get every bedroom in order. One set of drawers would be an amazing accomplishment. Get a babysitter for twice as long as you think you need, so if you finish early, you can put your feet up.

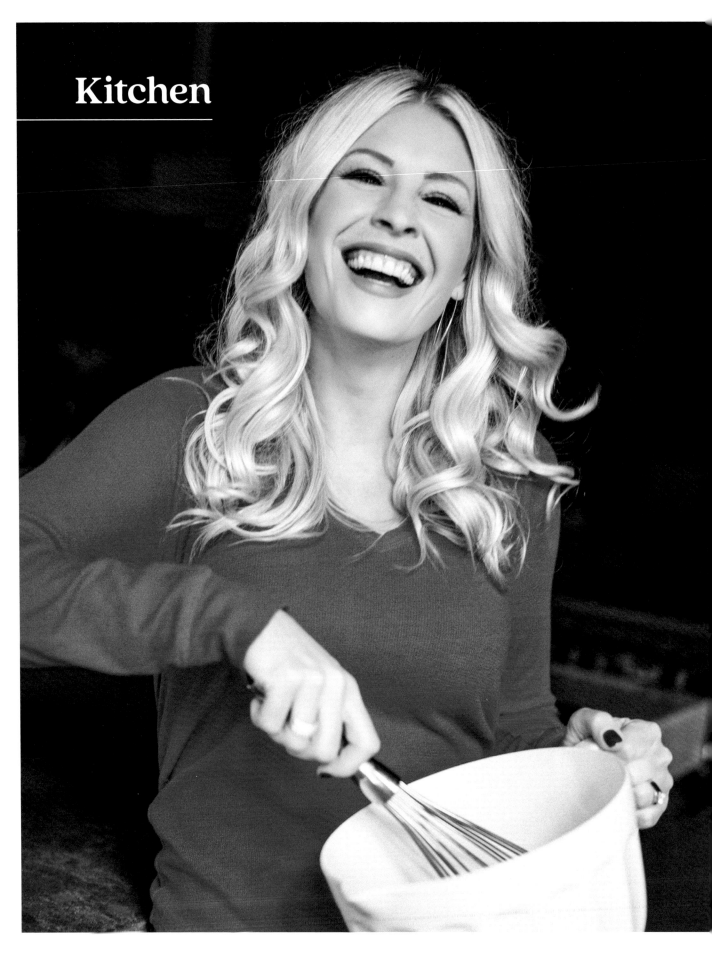

Kitchen

Deep breath! This is a big one, but you've got this. *And* it's incredibly rewarding to organize your kitchen. Also, remember that you don't have to do your whole kitchen at once (it's easier that way, though, if you're able to do it!). It's best to start when you have a few hours, and take on only what you're able to finish so you don't get overwhelmed.

The next few pages detail how I organize my kitchen with tips I've learned along the way. I've also included an inventory of my fridge and pantry in the Appendix (page 223) because I love when people share their ideas for healthy food/snacks and organization, so I'm sharing mine with you. I'll have items in my pantry that you'd never use, and vice versa! But hopefully, this section will give you some great ideas.

Okay, let's get started.

STEP 1: Take everything out that you're going to organize today.

STEP 2: Clean the shelves and drawers.

STEP 3: Organize the items into categories and make a pile to be given away.

STEP 4: Put categorized items together in containers.

I use clear, white, gray, or wooden containers; expandable trays; and interlocking organizer trays. Here, on the next few pages, is my system:

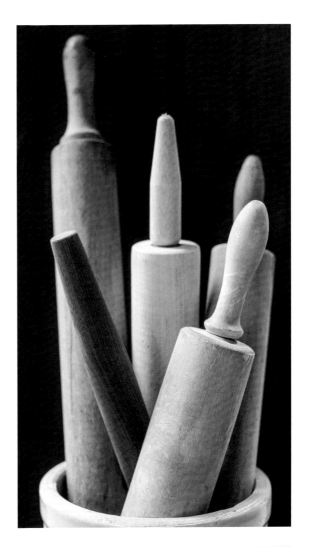

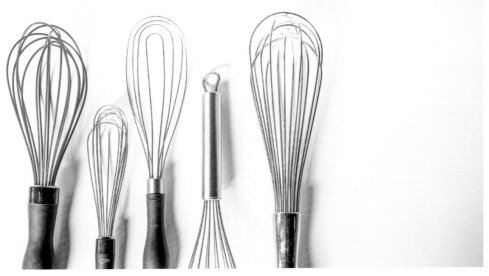

What Goes in Drawers

SILVERWARE: I keep all spoons, forks, knives, steak knives, and metal straws in the silverware drawer, closest to the table for easy setting. I also keep a lighter for lighting table candles along with toothpicks for finger foods in this drawer. For some reason, silverware drawers get crazy, becoming the catchall for everything from take-out chopsticks and red pepper packets to the random fork a friend left at your house. So, like any other drawer, take everything out, purge it, organize it, and put back only what you need. (Toss those red pepper packets or funnel them into your spice jar and return your friend's spoon.)

COOKING UTENSILS: Spatulas, whisks, wooden spoons, knives, tongs, and scissors. (I keep all my knives in a butcher block that fits *in* the drawer because I like to keep my countertop clutter-free.)

SERVING UTENSILS: Large serving spoons and forks, cheese knives, cheese markers, and pie servers.

BARBECUE UTENSILS: Barbecue tongs, spatulas, hamburger press, meat skewers, thermometers, and tenderizer mallet.

SHREDDING, SLICING, AND PEELING UTENSILS: Pizza slicer, cheese grater, egg slicer, peeler, mandoline, herb and kale stripper, corn stripper, and zester.

SCOOPING UTENSILS: Ladles, cookie scoops, ice cream scoops, metal cooking spoons.

MEASURING UTENSILS: Spoons, cups.

OPENERS, ET CETERA: Can opener, bottle opener, jar opener, pasta maker, fondue forks and skewers, drink muddler.

BAKING AND CANDY-MAKING SUPPLIES: Paper and silicone muffin pan liners, biscuit cutter, bench scraper, pie weights, candy thermometer, cake frosting tools, pastry blender, and silicone pot holders (I use only silicone, because cloth pot holders get ruined and look nasty quickly). When we built our house, we put in kick drawers to utilize the space under the cabinets. So this is where I store baking sheets and muffin tins, stacked by size. It's amazing how using that typically wasted space helps.

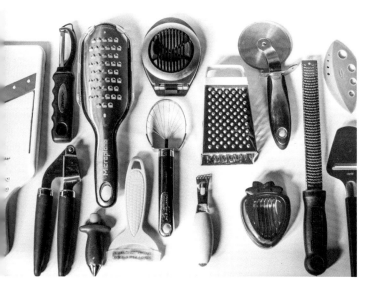

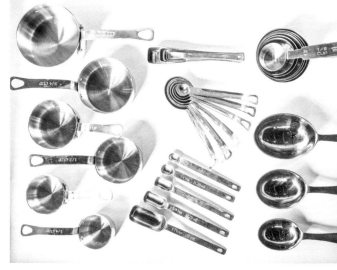

CUTTING BOARDS: I keep all cutting boards (wooden and plastic) together in one drawer, with the plastic ones on top since I use those the most. I oil the wooden boards frequently to keep them in good shape.

SPICES: Spices are my other love language! When organizing my friends' homes, I almost always start with their spices. Most people keep them in the cupboard, but I like to see everything, so I keep mine in a drawer. To start, I pour the store-bought spices into small glass jars using a funnel, put a label on top, and then alphabetize them. It makes cooking a lot faster! (I buy my spices in bulk and keep the large amounts in big mason jars, on the highest shelves of my cupboards, and then I just refill the small spice jars as needed.)

pro TIP If you don't have enough drawers in your kitchen to have each of these categories in their own individual drawer, you can use dividers to keep everything more organized.

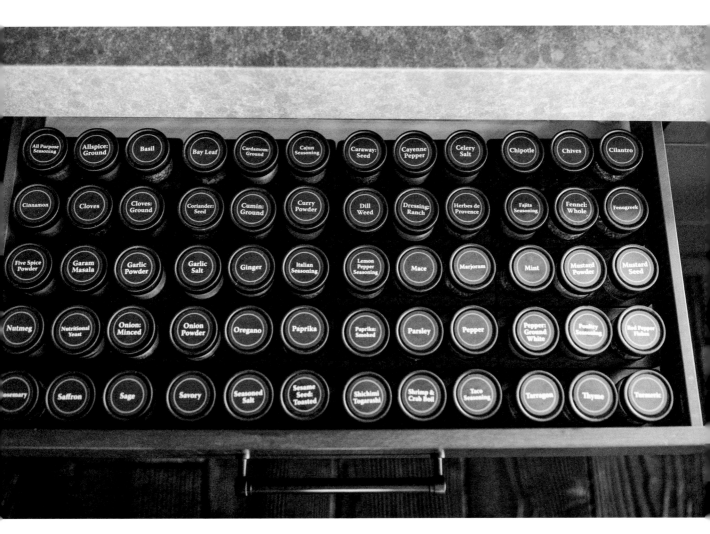

What Goes in Cabinets

DRINKWARE AND DISHWARE: I love my drinkware and dishware to be simple and uniform—as much as possible. We frequently purge cups, mugs, and water bottles (how do we collect four hundred of them?!); I have Brian and the kids pick their favorites and then I donate the rest. I keep the uniform dishware and drinkware in cabinets that are easily accessible. And because I don't like bright colors, logos, or patterns, I try to keep all that stuff in a separate cupboard or drawer that's not opened by guests.

KID WORLD: I keep the kid-ware simple. I use silicone suction plates, weighted straw sippy cups, and spill-proof snack holders. For my first babies, I bought every gadget and baby item possible, but the truth is, I didn't need that much. Because we make so many frozen fruit juice pops, we also have a storage bin for sticks and holders.

FOOD CONTAINERS: I have three sections of food containers with lids: glass for storing food in the fridge; plastic to-go containers for lunches (my kids can't take glass to school); and airtight containers for dry goods. Since plastic containers wear out, warp in the dishwasher, and often end up without a matching lid, this is a good area to purge frequently! About once a month, I go through backpacks, cars, and the dishwasher and lay out all the containers and their lids. If I can't find a matching lid or bottom, it gets donated. Don't think twice; just toss it. It's gone just like the missing sock you can't find. Let. It. Go.

DISPOSABLE PRODUCTS: I hate waste, but since we're constantly hosting people, I keep disposable products stocked so the dishes don't get crazier than they already are (sigh). I keep large and dessert-size paper plates, bowls, and cups; plastic utensils; paper napkins; and disposable straws in a drawer closest to the table.

APPLIANCES AND GADGETS: I feel like I own half of Williams-Sonoma because anyone who knows me knows that I *love* cooking and cooking gadgets. Food is pretty much my only hobby. Ha! Every birthday or Christmas for twenty-one years I've added to my collection. I love anything that can make preparing food faster and easier (like how I use my food processor with the shredding attachment to grate a block of cheese in two seconds instead of ten minutes and also without grating my knuckles). When I buy an appliance (or anything, really!), I try to buy it in a neutral color because most people get tired of bright-colored things after a few years.

If you have a side spot, like a walk-in pantry with a door, you can station large and noisy appliances for use in there—like blenders and espresso makers. It keeps things more streamlined and quieter in the main kitchen area, especially in the morning! When we remodeled, we turned our old tiny kitchen into a little prep kitchen for this reason.

I like to keep my kitchen appliances, gadgets, and containers in my kitchen cabinets, rather than have them on the countertops. I'm a sucker for empty

 pro TIP As you go through your drawers and cabinets and find things that you don't use, aren't in great condition, or are not a complete set (like measuring cups/ spoons), donate them or discard!

counters! So I keep all colanders, strainers, funnels, mixer attachments, baking dishes and pie pans, mixing bowls with lids, and other gadgets hidden in the cabinets, in an organized fashion, of course.

CLEANING PRODUCTS: We keep all of our housecleaning products under the sink (unless we have toddlers; then they're kept out of reach), including dishwasher detergent, dishwasher rinse aid, dish soap, hand soap, and cleaners for countertops, wood, carpet, upholstery, windows, and stain remover (with five kids, stain remover is my best friend).

From the food we eat to beauty products, candles, and cleaning products—we avoid harmful chemicals in everything we use. So I try to purchase all-natural and nontoxic products as much as possible. I don't like to use sponges (because they hold so much bacteria), so I use cloth towels and paper towels. I buy everything I can in bulk to save money. For instance, I use bulk natural hand soap (to fill my glass soap dispensers in the kitchen and bathrooms) and bulk laundry detergent (to refill my large glass jar).

COFFEE AND TEA: Ahhhh, coffee . . . my love language. Thank You, Jesus! I keep all the coffee and tea items near each other in a little coffee/tea station and I store mugs and travel cups nearby. In our house, because we host so much and everyone has their favorite method, we have several coffee-making tools: an espresso machine and grinder, a Keurig, a pour-over set, a kettle, a regular coffee grinder, and a normal coffeepot for gatherings. I store coffee beans and Keurig pods in large glass containers.

For tea, I take the packets out of the box and organize all the tea bags in an expandable tray. That way when I'm hosting, I can just pull the tray out and put it on the counter near the kettle. It looks pretty, and people can easily choose which tea they want and make their own. I store loose-leaf tea in labeled glass containers.

When we remodeled, we also put a mini fridge in the prep kitchen, under the coffee/tea area, for quick access to all of our milk choices (almond, coconut, cow, oat, etc.). I also keep the coffee syrup in the mini fridge, so ants don't get into it. I *hate* ants.

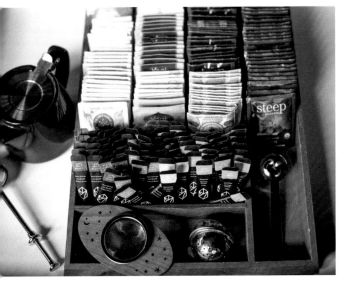
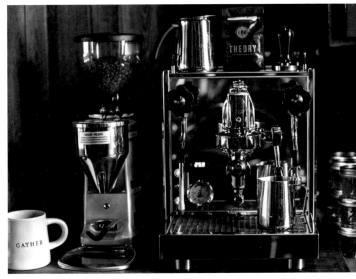

Room by Room

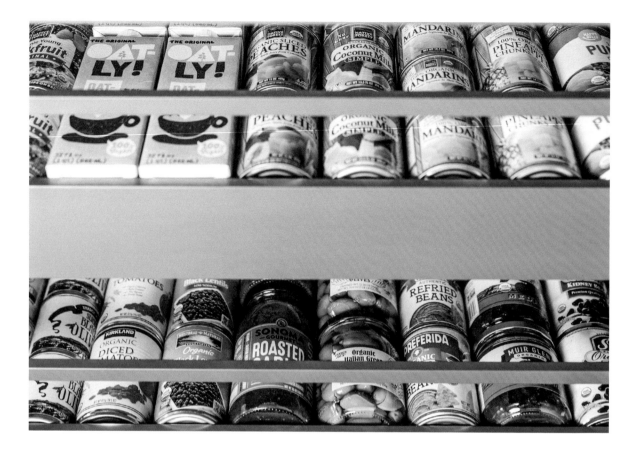

What Goes in the Pantry

Containers and pantries—a match made in heaven. If you don't have any airtight containers, I recommend getting a big box of them (I love the OXO brand and they're cheaper in a big box than individually) so you're ready for a pantry makeover. They will keep your food fresh longer, which means . . . you'll save money. But if you don't have any, like I said at the beginning, just use what you have for now and invest in the airtight later.

To start organizing, take all the food out of your pantry, cupboards, and drawers. Yes, it will be a mess, but it's the best way. Check the date of each item, toss anything expired, then group together "like items." Here's how I group mine:

CANNED GOODS: I keep in a drawer and separate them by sweet and savory.

OILS AND VINEGARS: Are organized in clear bins.

LIQUID SWEETENERS (HONEY, AGAVE NECTAR, MOLASSES): Are in a clear bin.

In airtight containers:

- Rice, lentils, and pasta.

- Baking ingredients.

- Breakfast foods (oatmeal, Cream of Wheat, cereal, dry smoothie ingredients).

- Opened snacks. (Never put the opened bag of snacks or cereal into the pantry. If they're not in an airtight container, you might as well toss them. No one wants to eat stale food.)

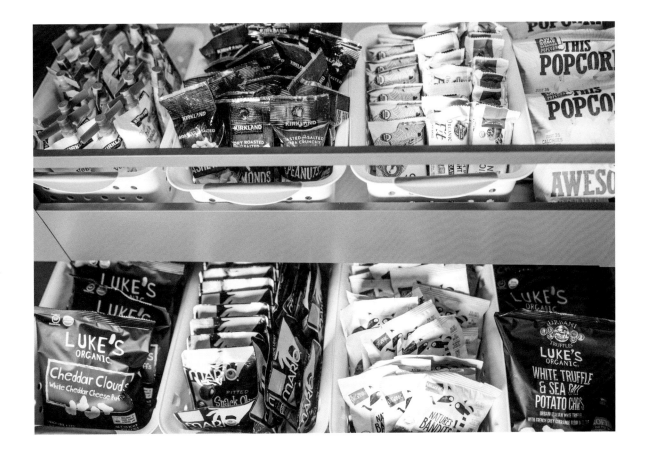

I store everything in clear containers and I use a label only if it's not apparent what the ingredient is—or if I need to note an expiration date. For example, I don't label cereal, but I label gluten-free flour with its expiration date. If you love labels, knock yourself out! I just don't like removing and replacing stickers when the contents change. For the items I do label, I put the label on the bottom of the container, so it doesn't show. I like the container faces to all look clean and uniform when I open the cupboard.

I also downsize my containers as the contents decrease, like cereal and snack food. I'm amazed at how my kids avoid eating an item if there's only a little left in a big container, but if it's in a downsized container, it's a quicker pick. Weird but tested and true. And I store only dry goods in the airtight containers because then I can switch them out easily without washing them.

For an entire inventory of what I keep in my pantry, see What's in My Kitchen (page 220).

SNACK DRAWER: I have a large pullout drawer in a lower cabinet for keeping healthy snacks accessible. If you don't have pullout drawers, just organize the snacks in bins on a shelf within kid reach. This is incredibly helpful for parents, because your kids can help themselves and also pack their own lunches at a young age. Praise.

I keep reusable silicone bags on hand for to-go snacks but only for the older kids. The little ones lose just about *everything*, and the reusable bags are expensive compared to the clear plastic bags.

Room by Room

What Goes in the Refrigerator

I organize my fridge contents into these groupings:

- Drinks
- Fruits
- Vegetables
- Dairy
- Vegan items
- PBJ
- Condiments and dressings
- Prepped food (chopped veggies and fruits or cooked meat)
- Meats and eggs
- Leftovers

Contain your items, like fruits and vegetables, in stackable containers with lids or pullout drawers to give you more room in your fridge.

I'm a major online shopper, so deliveries of most of my kitchen staples and snacks are on monthly subscriptions (for ease and savings with Amazon). As you're organizing your fridge, it's a great time to take note of the staples you're out of or running low on. I try to keep a backup of most things I buy so I don't run out. When I use the backup item, I order a new one to replace it. Grocery delivery is another godsend in our house, and the cost works out to be about the same as a membership to a bulk goods store—so I canceled my yearly membership to the bulk goods store and got a yearly delivery service (cheaper than paying each time). It saves a lot of time, and time is precious. (If you also calculate how much money you can make working an extra hour instead of making the trip to and from the grocery store every week, it's even more worth it.) Plus, it allows for flexibility and ease. I can order groceries when we are out of town and they are there when we get home—one of my favorite time-savers.

See What's in My Kitchen (page 220) for an inventory of my refrigerator to give you healthy food ideas and the Food Storage Guide (page 223) for tips on storing food to help you get the most for your money with organic food!

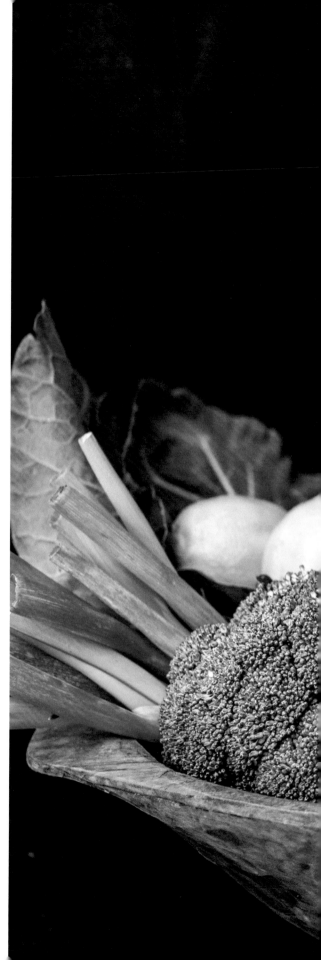

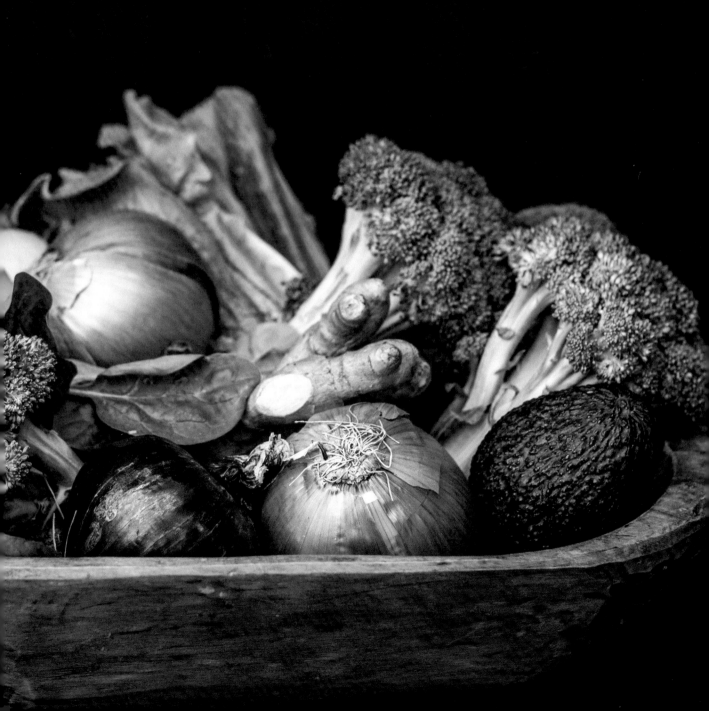

pro TIP To make your fridge look amazing, dump the contents of items (like a huge jar of pickles) into large clear mason jars. I know, I know, this is very next-level. But it's *so* lovely.

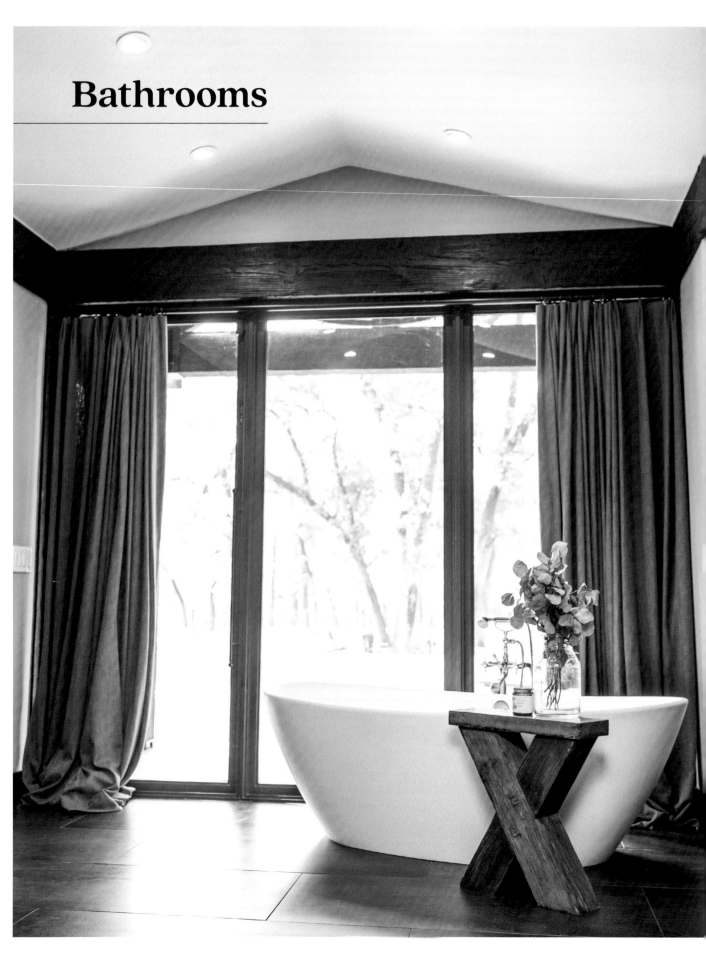

Bathrooms

To start organizing your bathroom, bring in empty containers and two trash bags. First, pull everything out of the drawers and cupboards and place those items on the floor. Although it is a big mess initially, in the end it makes it easier than doing it drawer by drawer and cupboard by cupboard. Next, wipe out the drawers and shelves with an all-purpose cleaner. Then start grouping all the items that go together. Make two separate piles: one for trash and one for giveaway—a garbage bag for each works great. Remember, get rid of it if you don't need it or if you don't love it. The lotions or perfume you can't stand the smell of? Give them away! Use the items that only have a little bit left in them first (from multiple containers of lotions or toothpastes, for example) so you free up more space in your bathroom.

I categorize our bathroom like this:

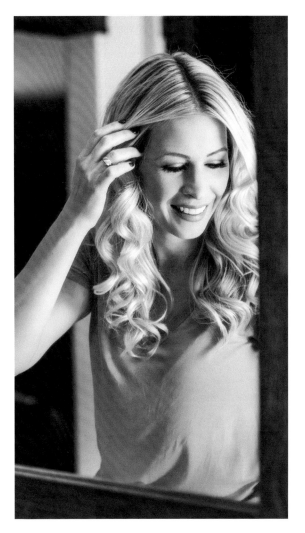

- **Teeth** (toothbrushes, toothbrush chargers, toothpaste, floss, whitening strips).

- **Shaving** (razors, blades, shaving cream, trimmers).

- **Hair** (hairbrushes, hair ties, combs, hair products, hair tools).

- **Nails** (nail clippers, nail files, polish, polish remover, cotton pads).

- **Face** (lotion, makeup and brushes, tweezers, eyelash curler, makeup remover wipes).

- **Bath and shower** (Epsom salts, bath bombs, bar soaps, scrubs, shampoos, conditioners).

- **Medical** (over-the-counter pain meds, allergy meds, cold meds, personal meds, wound care).

- **Deodorant and cologne.**

- **Body lotion.**

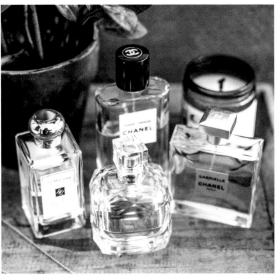

"By going through every room in your house,
getting rid of the junk, and organizing,
you'll not only have more space in your home,
but you'll also have more space emotionally."

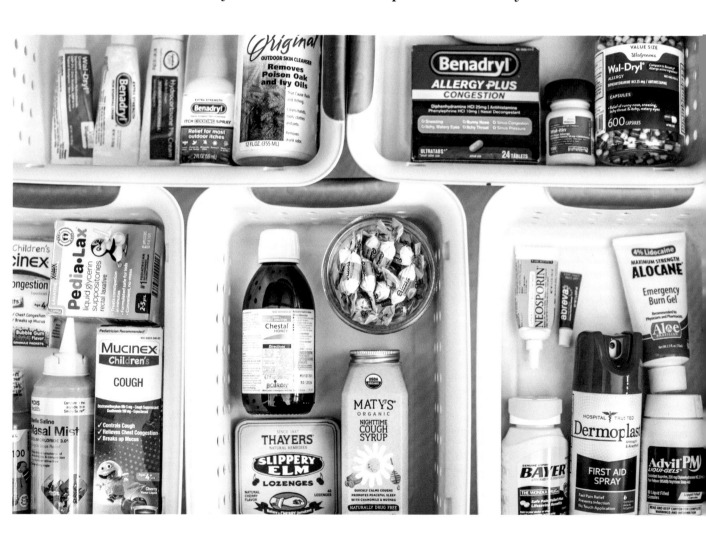

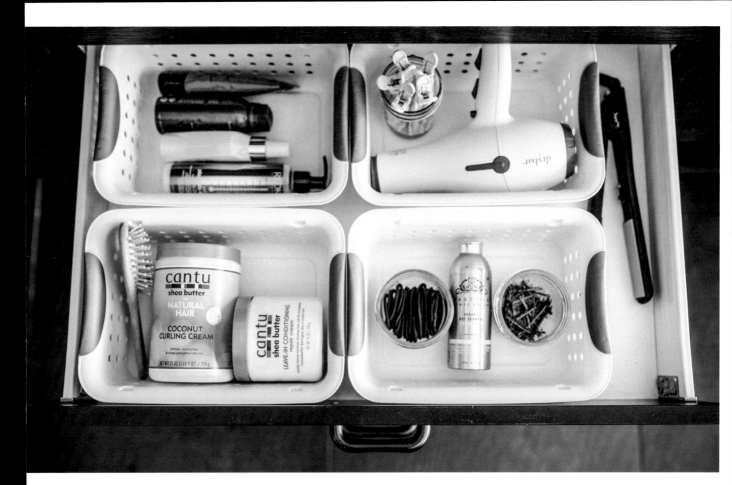

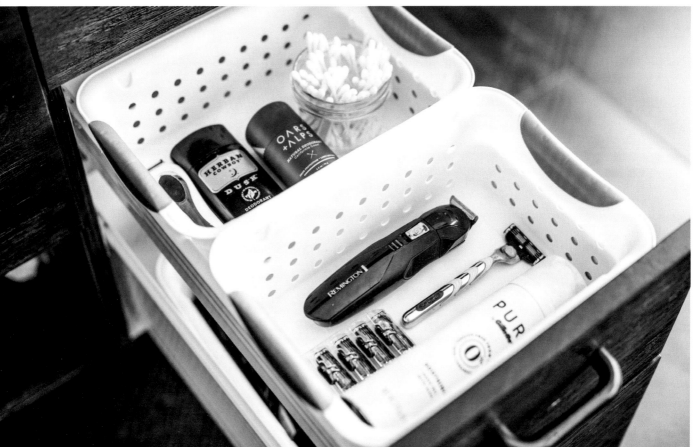

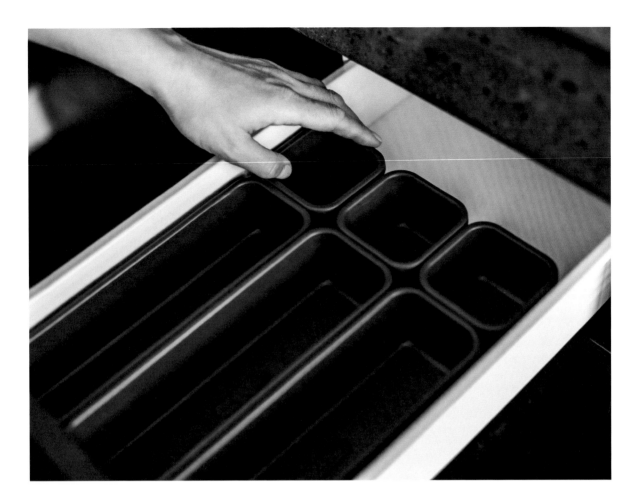

Usually, I put dental, shaving, and face items in drawers. I also place deodorant, cologne, and body lotion in drawers. But hair, nails, bath/shower, and medical stuff goes in cabinets. Each category has its own container, so it's easy to pull one out when needed, put it away after use, and still remain organized.

Sometimes, if you're like us, you'll realize that your bathroom has a junk drawer. I don't know how it happens or what kind of demonic force causes it, but Brian's bathroom drawer needs constant help. I find any and everything in there. It's like a magnet for all his worlds . . . guitar picks, screwdrivers, knives, bullets, and his toothbrush. (Face palm.) It's all stuff he wants to keep; it's just not where it should go! But since he's fallen in love with organization over the years, and knows how much I

care about it, I usually just give that junk drawer the eye . . . and we both tackle it.

For a guest bathroom (ours gets used daily), you won't have as many personal care products in those drawers, but I try to keep as many personal items as I can think of that a guest would need when visiting (cologne/perfume, bandages, dental floss, over-the-counter pain reliever, etc.) in the drawers for their convenience. You can point the guests toward the guest bathroom when they need something instead of running around the house in the middle of a party trying to help them. I also stock a few fresh hand towels, extra soap, toilet paper, and cleaning supplies and paper towels under the sink in case there's a mess. Plus, I love how anticipating the needs of guests makes them feel comfortable, taken care of, and at home . . . hospitality at its finest.

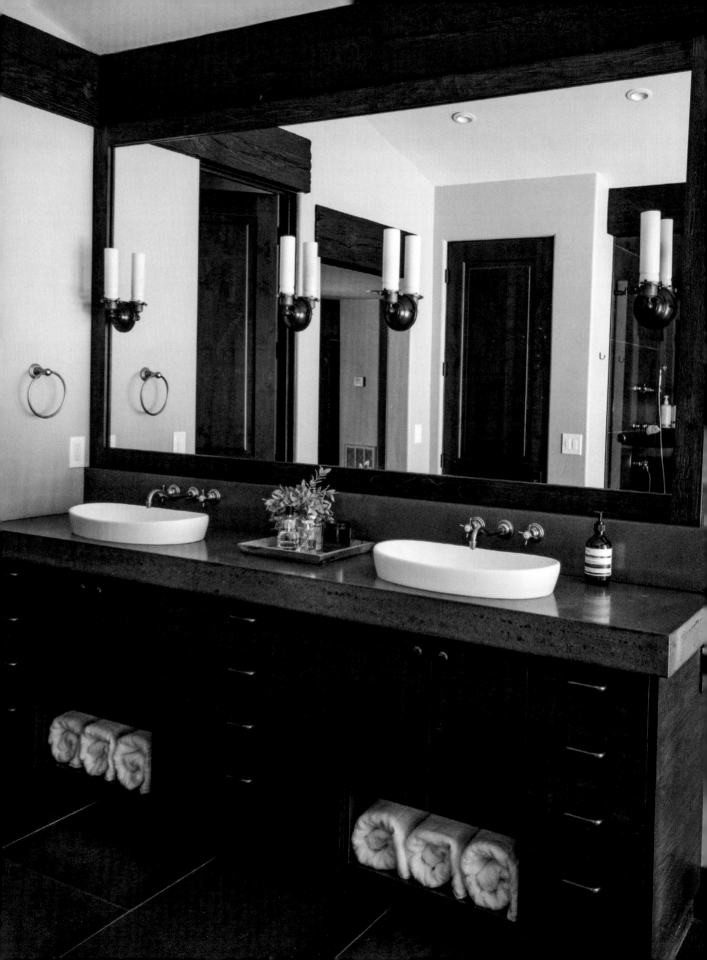

Home Office

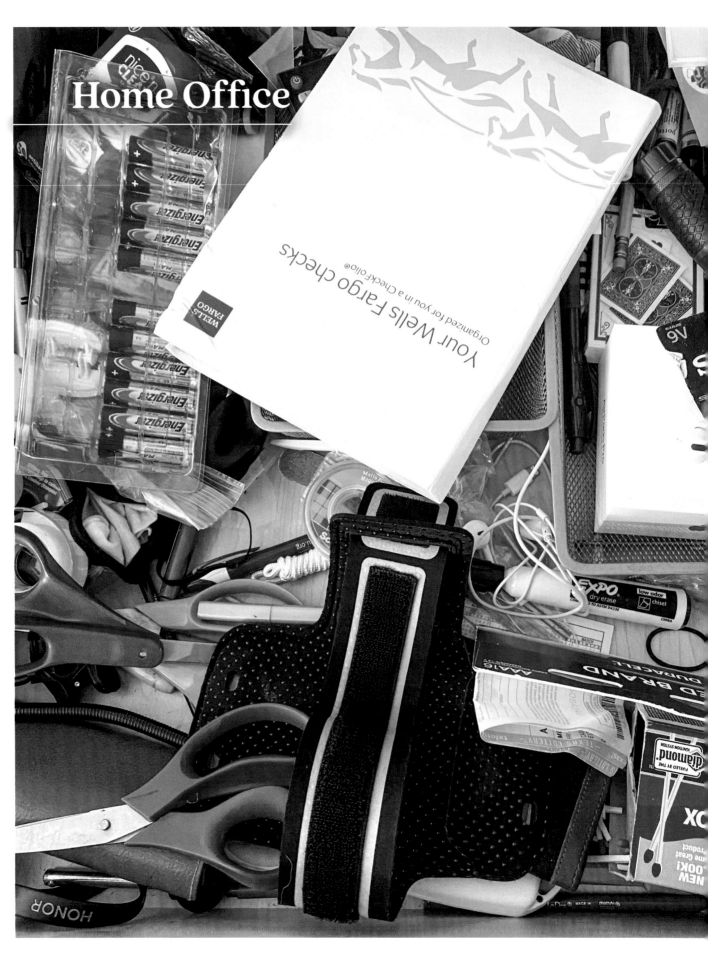

Being writers and having a lot of kids with schoolwork means our desks are well used! So keeping our office and school supplies stocked and organized really makes life easier for us.

Most people (especially if you have kids) have pens, pencils, crayons, and markers scattered throughout their entire house. Step 1 is to go through your whole house and collect all the stragglers (this is a great chore for kids or helpful friends). Put them on the kitchen table and start by tossing any crayons or pencils that are broken or in bad shape. Next check the pens on scrap paper to see which ones are full of ink. Iffy? Toss them. Then set the "in good condition" items on the counter, have everyone pick their favorites—and then take them back to their desks. For things like paper clips, do you really need a thousand? In my lifetime, I'll probably use twenty. Give away the rest! Remember, space in your home is precious.

I used to feel bad about tossing all our half-used crayons, so I bought a wax-melting machine to repurpose them. It was a huge mess, and it went to Goodwill the next day! I hate wasting, but some things simply aren't worth keeping, and a worn-out crayon is one of them. Your kids will have hundreds of them as they get new ones every year in grade school. *Let them go.*

In addition to these normal desk and school items, I also keep a binder of our family's important documents in one folder so I can easily grab them in case of a fire. Birth certificates, adoption papers, passports, shot records, vehicle titles—all in one place. For our photos, we keep those backed up on hard drives and store them in a fireproof safe.

Something I purge often? Email! (There's no way email is going to be in heaven—it's the worst!) On a weekly basis, I weed through my emails and immediately unsubscribe from any junk that's coming through. (Just open the email, scroll to the bottom of it, and hit that beautiful "unsubscribe" link.) I also have a second email I use when I don't want to use my personal one (like when we're buying a car or online shopping); it helps your personal email have less junk.

The Actual Junk Drawer!

Everyone has a junk drawer or . . . many junk drawers. The keeper of batteries, expired coupons, rubber bands, mysterious keys, loose change, bag clips, scissors, twist ties, safety pins, receipts from five years ago, countless pens, and for our family a million guitar picks. It's like you're always ready to play (and dominate) that game at summer camp: "The first person to run onstage with this item wins!"

The junk drawer requires constant upkeep to stay organized because it's just too easy to throw something in that drawer and walk away. But take a minute and put the item where it belongs. I've probably spent sixty percent of my life the past fifteen years putting things back where they belong. It's maddening at times, but I just love it when someone is looking for something, and instead of searching high and low for it, I can just tell them exactly where it is. Ahhh. . . . the reward . . . it's lovely.

The way to start organizing a junk drawer is to identify what *should* be in this drawer. In our house, we have two drawers for most of these items. In one drawer we keep batteries, flashlights, lighters, utility candles, matches (we know right where to go in case of a power outage), a measuring tape, glue, and a small tool kit for projects in the house. In the other drawer we keep everything related to electronics: computer and phone chargers, headphones, screen protectors, and portable speakers. Everything else gets put away where it should go and that's the end of the junk drawer.

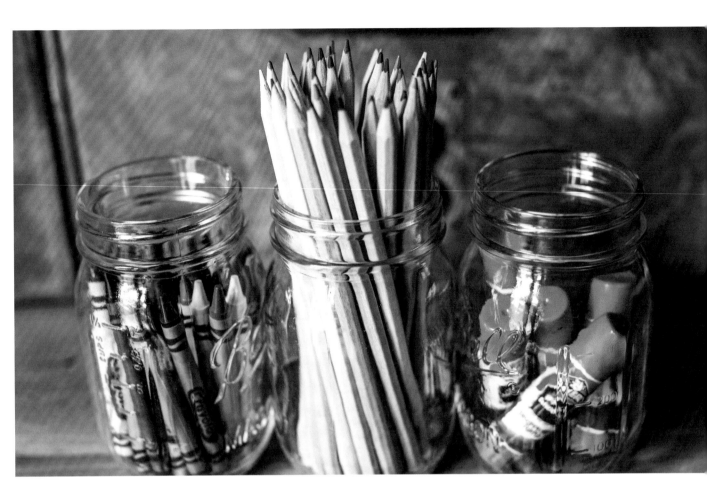
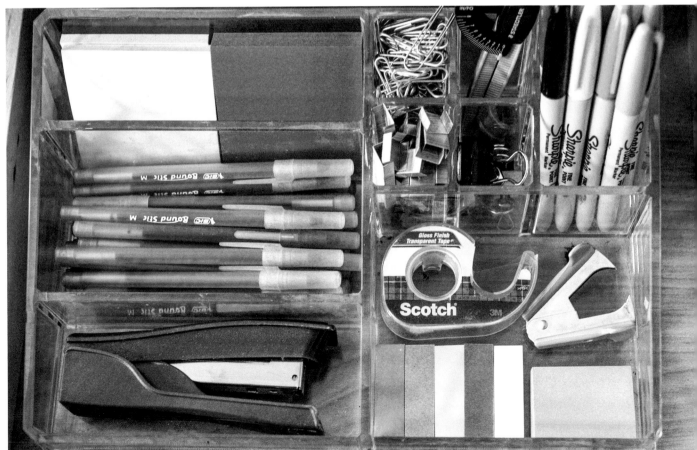

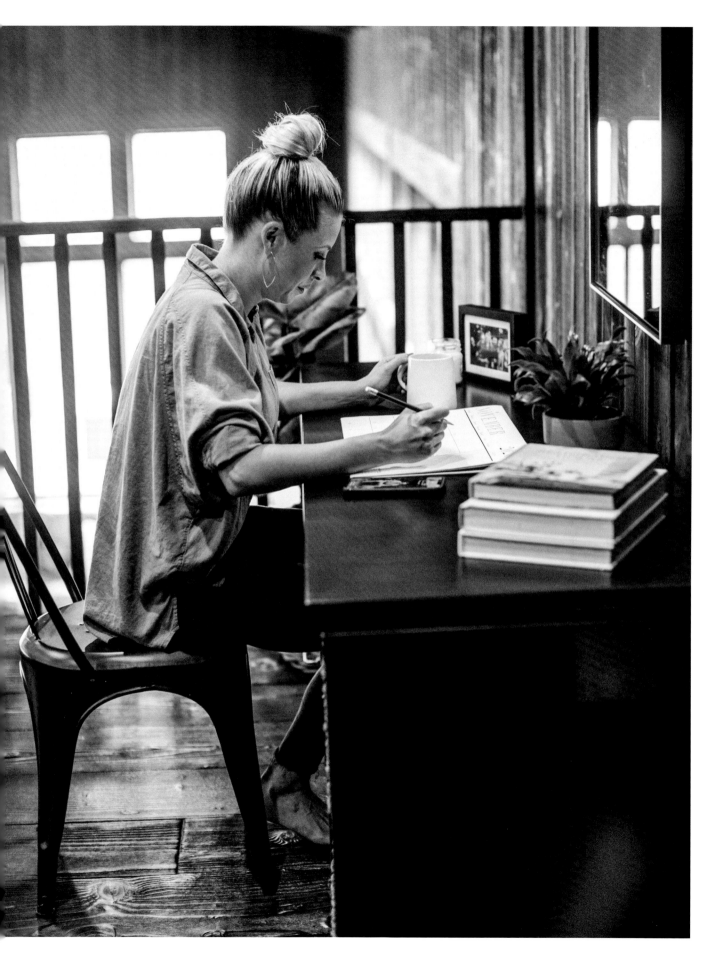

Closets

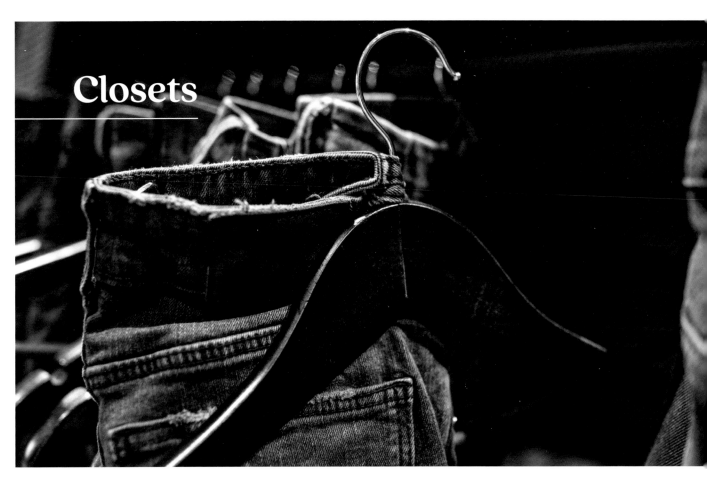

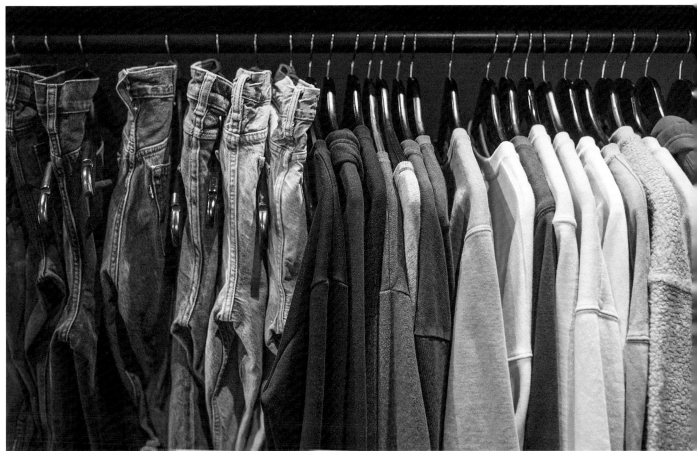

Like most people, you probably have clothes in your closet that aren't in style, don't fit well, or have never looked great on you in the first place. (Many times emotional "junk" gets dealt with as you work through your clothes.) So when I'm organizing and purging my clothes closet, I get help from friends who have great style and can help me purge/keep/ know what to buy next time. It helps to have your friends be honest about what looks good and what needs to go! Instead of holding on to "pipe-dream" clothes for someday, let those go to somebody who can wear them today. Give yourself permission to *let them go*.

The coat you got as a present that you haven't removed the tag from because you don't even like it? Give it away or sell it. The shirt your mom loves on you, but you hate? Yep, you guessed it . . . give it away or sell it. And as a general guideline, if you haven't worn it in a year, you probably never will . . . so get rid of it. Have you put on weight and your clothes are too tight? Who hasn't?! Don't hate yourself for where you're at right now. Make some fitness and good health commitments today, but wear clothes that fit you great now and be okay with it. That's right . . . let those "when I was skinny" jeans go.

Here's the deal:

Closets should not hold our guilt, our obligations, or our false realities . . . Yes, that will PREACH!

Don't worry about having nothing left. You'll be okay, I promise. And the simplicity will bring you peace and joy when you step into your closet. Because I can tell you from personal experience, it's *amazing* to walk into your purged closet, now filled with in-style clothes that all fit you great!

I keep things minimal as much as possible, except for my twenty-plus black T-shirts (my tour uniform; you never know if you'll be able to do laundry so I bring a lot). Always slimming, don't show sweat, always in style . . . I'm a practical girl! I

like classic, timeless pieces and I can't stand trying too hard. I just want to be comfortable and modest. So it's jeans and a T-shirt most days for me, with some cozy layers and a few nicer things for events and date nights.

In my closet, I hang most of my clothes—it's easiest to see what I have at a glance—and I keep them grouped like this: tank tops, short-sleeved shirts, long-sleeved shirts, sweaters, coats, robes, dresses, jeans, dress pants, and bags.

Directly on my closet shelves, I store shoes with their heels facing out and organized by style: flats, heels, boots, sandals, and athletic shoes. I have a step stool tucked away close by to help reach the high shelves.

In baskets on my shelves, I keep loose items categorized like this:

Underwear
Everyday socks
Cozy socks
Everyday bras
Strapless and sports bras
Slips and undergarments
Lingerie
Leggings
Sweats
Hats
Clutches

If you have a dresser rather than shelves, I recommend investing in some drawer dividers and separating your items similarly. If you need more storage space, a door rack is a great solution for keeping hats and bags organized and in one place (I recommend keeping it inside your closet for a cleaner look in your bedroom).

I also have a basket in my closet for mismatched socks, which I despise, but alas . . . it is life. Every few months I check for lost matches behind the dryer and in the car, then throw away any I can't pair up. You just have to toss them. (But seriously, where the heck do they go?!)

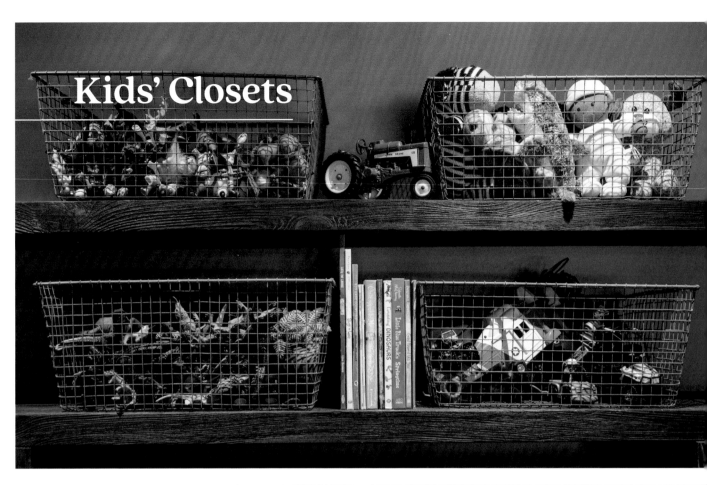

Kids' Closets

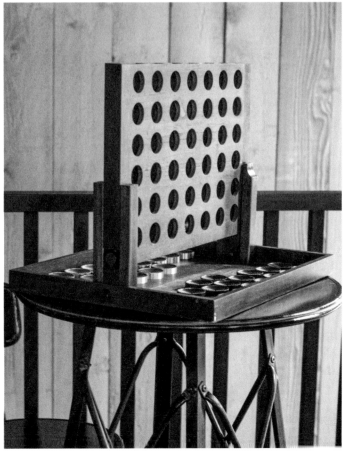

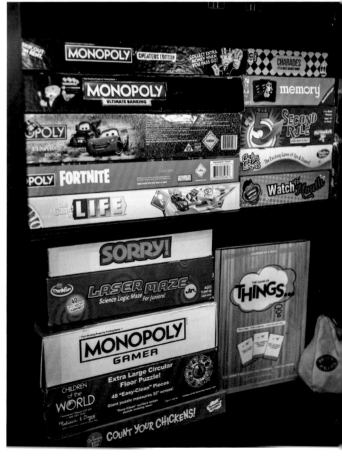

Kids grow out of and wear out their clothes fast! For that reason, I go through all their clothes and shoes at least twice a year. I make two piles: one for giveaway and one for the "save for younger sibling" box in storage. If there's no younger sibling, it all goes to the "giveaway" pile. Often, when I have something to give away, the Holy Spirit will bring someone to mind so I'll send them a text to see if they can use it. It's pretty amazing how often it's just what they need! Such a beautiful way to love your community! Many times in my life, people have given to me in this way and it was amazing!

All the Toys

Toys multiply crazy-fast, and my younger kids are always bringing home the most random things from school and birthday parties! I keep all the little kids' toys organized in containers by themes (at left), and we let them play with one theme at a time. Before they get out something else, I have them clean up what they're playing with. I've noticed that my kids enjoy and play with their toys *way* more this way than when it's chaotic.

I keep the containers of toys and games up on a high shelf that only an adult can reach. When they're ready for a new toy theme, they clean up and I swap containers. For cards and games, the boxes they come in usually get trashed, so I put them in containers or bags once their boxes start to fall apart. I love clear containers for all of this stuff so you can see what's in them.

Because we don't like toys spread all over the house, we designate ninety percent of the toys to one play area. I keep most of our toddler's toys in my closet so he can play with them while I get ready and do laundry; he also has a play kitchen set in our great room. We didn't do a designated toy area when we first had kids, and it was nuts! Ten years later, we got smarter. Our toddler, Ryder, has an amazing sense

of cleaning up, and he usually does it without fussing because he's just been raised in this "clean up before you get more toys" model. Even if your kids are older, it's worth making this part of the daily routine.

There are thousands of toy themes so I don't separate everything, but I do categorize them as much as possible like this:

Vehicles (cars, trucks, tractors, etc.)
Dinosaurs and animals
Blocks, LEGO sets, and Lincoln Logs
Puzzles and games
Books
Stuffed animals and characters (Disney, Marvel, etc.)
Play food/kitchen
Dolls and dress-up
Art supplies
Outdoor toys and sports equipment

Stuffed animals pile up (and get gross) so I have my kids keep out only their ten favorites and we purge frequently. Most stuffed animals can't be washed, and anything that can't be washed gets nasty.

Another thing that will help to keep your toy world streamlined is to register your kids online for birthdays and Christmas. That way, they get only the stuff they'll play with (parents know best), *and* your friends and family won't waste good money on something that they already have or something that gets used only once and breaks. It's also how we've built on our set collections (i.e., LEGOs, Littlest Pet Shop and accessories, toy kitchen accessories/toy food) and avoided duplicates. And then they'll play with the other part of their collection that they already have more!

For outdoor toys and sports equipment, we keep it all categorized in the garage. If one of the kids outgrows their soccer cleats, I sell them or give them away. Keeping them in case the next kid plays soccer rarely works and it's just more clutter in your house you don't need. Get rid of them!

Keep only favorites.

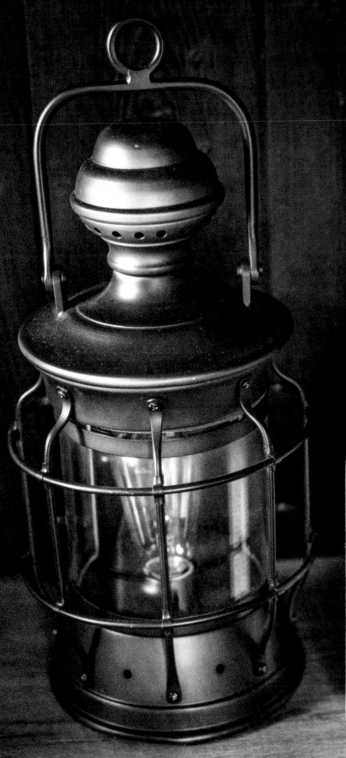
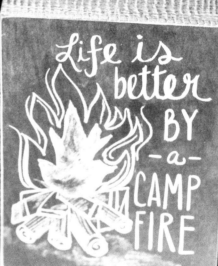

Life is
better
BY
-a-
CAMP
FIRE

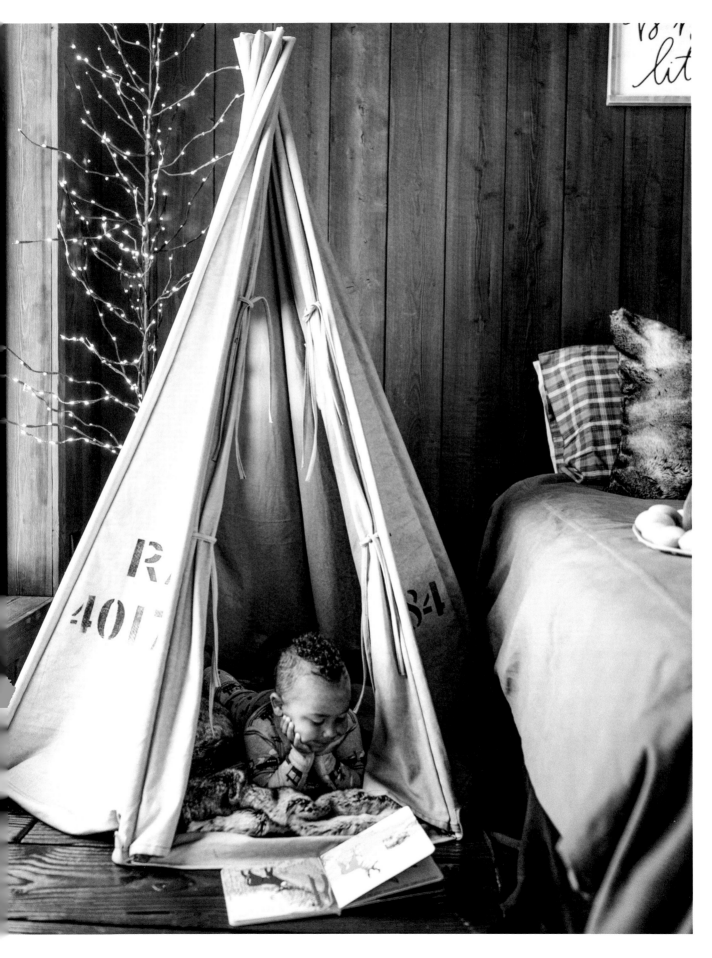

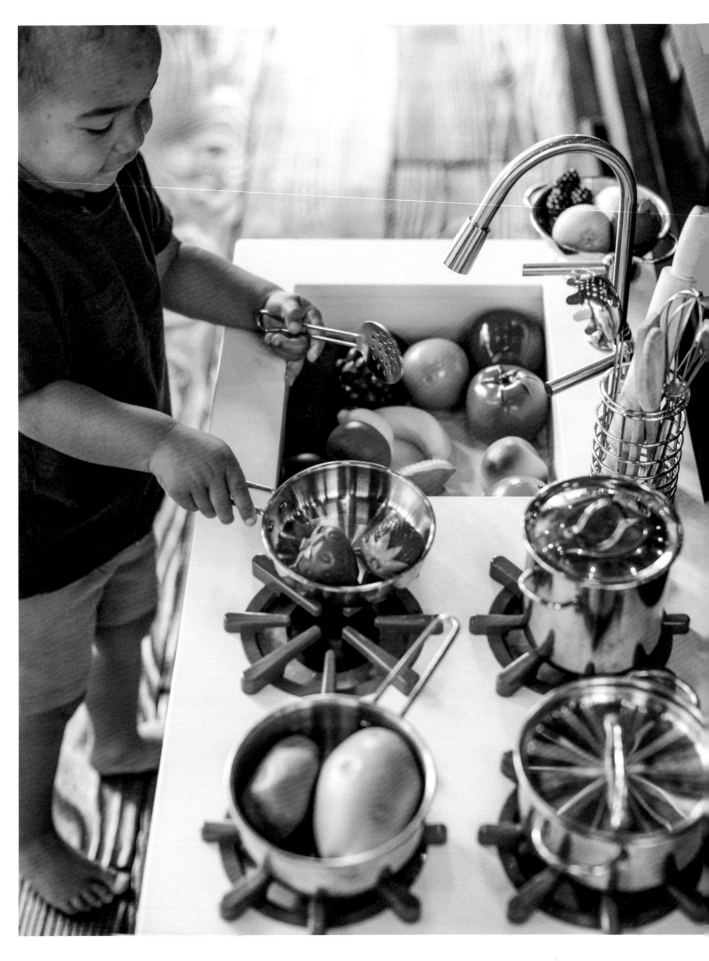

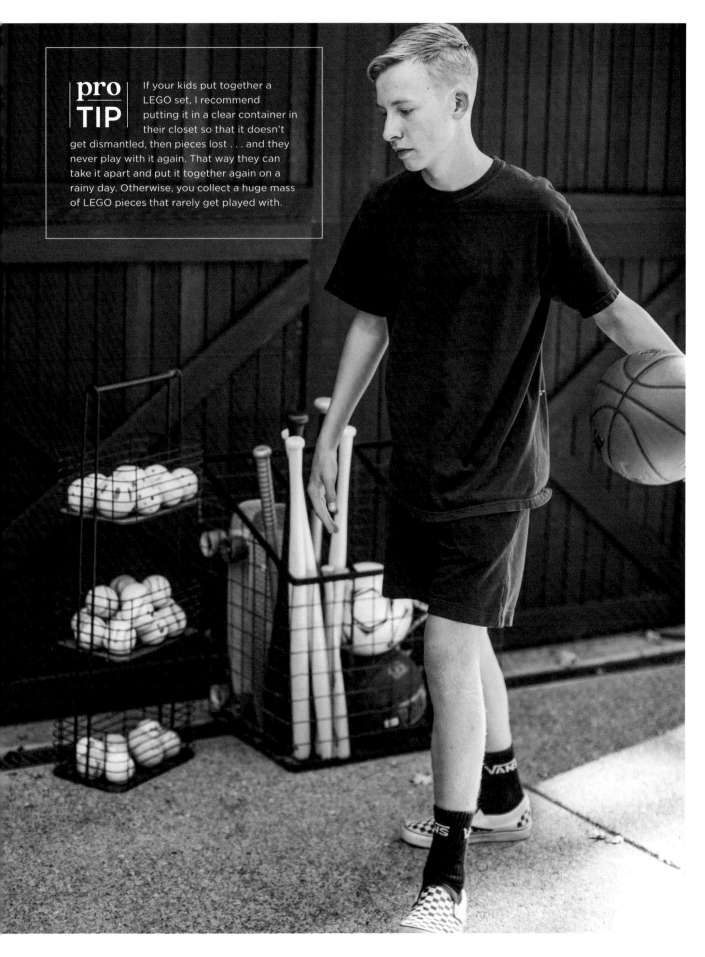

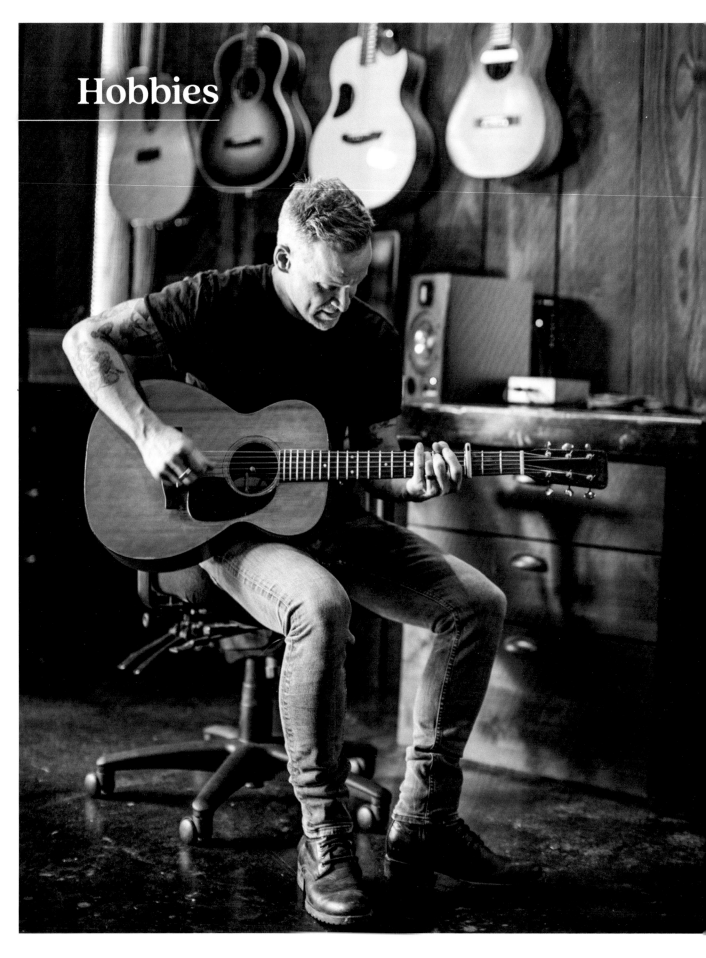

Hobbies

I could have titled this section "Brian Land," since he's the hobbyist in our family. (I mean, technically, my hobby is food and kitchen gadgets, but I don't think that counts.) You probably have one or more of your own hobby lovers in the house—and maybe it's you!

Brian has had *sooooo* many hobbies over the twenty-one years we've been together, and there tends to be so much stuff that goes along with them. Guitars, studio equipment, fishing, bows, beekeeping, raising chickens, raising goats, guns, camping, backpacking, and more. One year he bought all the equipment for hatching quail eggs, and then once they hatched, our cats ate them all . . . Oh, the circle of life. There was also the time he had a massive fish tank and a ball python. Sick! At first, putting structure around these hobbies took a lot of effort. But now we have everything organized in large containers in the barn. And, thankfully, he has streamlined his hobbies over the years so now there are a few less.

No matter what your hobbies are, keep them purged, organized, and in labeled containers in the garage, attic, or storage unit. They don't need to take up valuable space inside your home unless you're using them every day.

Keepsakes

The best way I've found to handle this one is for each person in the family to have their own container that holds everything that is special to them from childhood to present day. For my sentimental children, their boxes are bigger than mine or Brian's. When our kids are little, I know there's a lot of "Save every little scrap of paper they've colored on," but it's best to just save the ones that stand out. I don't think anyone's ever looked back on their childhood stuff and thought, *Wow, I'm glad I have two hundred pieces of paper with preschool watercolors.* Give the art its moment on the fridge, and then toss it. Save only the stuff that matters.

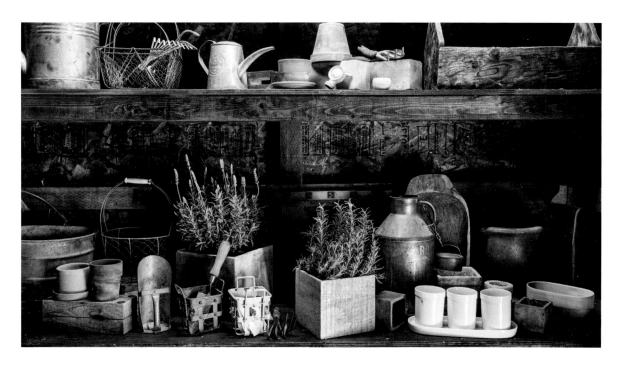

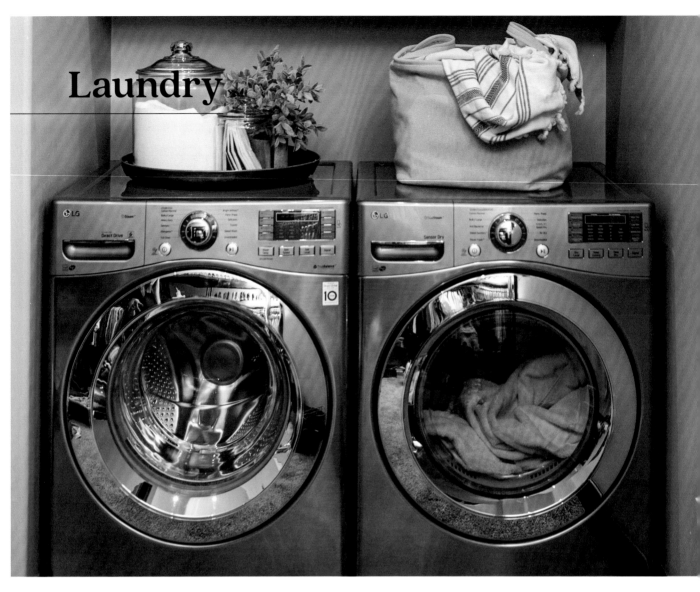

Laundry

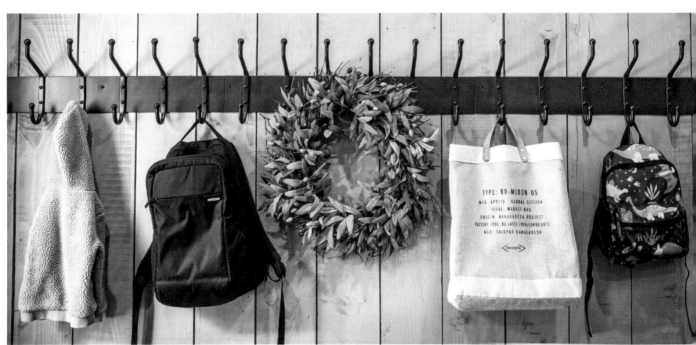

Laundry and the love of God are the same . . . never ending.

I keep a tray on top of my dryer with laundry detergent, stain spray, dryer sheets, starch spray, a lint roller, and bleach. (I try to keep products as natural as possible, but sometimes you just need some bleach . . . amen?) Keeping these products contained in a wicker basket, tray, or cabinet makes the chore of doing laundry feel less chaotic and more intentional. I also have a "Scripture of the Day" paper that I keep on my dryer, since I seem to live in my laundry area and it's a great time to meditate on the Word!

When we were building our house, I saw a picture on Pinterest of a washer and dryer in a couple's closet. I thought, *That is genius!* It made so much sense—no need for a laundry room, just a spacious closet! So we put a tile floor in our closet for the washer and dryer, and not carting huge laundry baskets around has changed our lives. Clothes come off and into the laundry when we change and we pull them out of the dryer to hang them up. In the first phase of remodeling our house we had the washer and dryer in our closet so the kids had to bring their laundry down and pack it up to their rooms. A few years later we were able to build a second mini laundry area (with a stackable washer and dryer) upstairs in a hall closet where the kids now do their own laundry, and they don't have to be in our master bedroom space every day. It's amazing for all. If you can manage to have a second laundry space, I would recommend it!

Mudroom or House Entryway

Whether you have an entryway or an actual mudroom, every house needs a place where you can contain all those shoes, backpacks, and bags. It's a daily opportunity to restore order! Like any common area, our family feels more at peace when those places are organized and not just a dumping ground.

As much as possible, we don't wear shoes inside the house (because God knows what is on those shoes). We have a bench in our mudroom area with three drawers for shoes. (When we built the house we only had three kids, a drawer for each, but we've added two more babies! At least their shoes are tiny for the time being.) We also installed metal hooks for backpacks, coats, and dog leashes. Since we live on a farm, rubber boots are a huge part of our lives, so we built an area just for boots too.

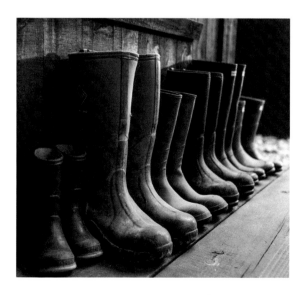

Garage and Storage

I try to keep our garage as clutter-free as possible, but it still holds a large toolbox, a small gym, two freezers, all the kids' sporting equipment, two strollers, bicycles, skateboards, and more. We don't keep cars in the garage because we love having the extra space to use as an indoor/outdoor playroom for the kids, especially on rainy days. And besides, I'd like to keep my car as scratch-free as possible when my kids are using the garage as their own personal skatepark.

When we built our garage, we added a storage room off to the side. Since we host an event almost every week at our house, we needed a place to hold all those event supplies like vases, candles, platters, glassware, large charcuterie boards, party decor, seasonal decor, wreaths, present boxes, wrapping paper, gift bags, and more! Depending on how much you entertain, this type of collection could also go in bins in the garage or in a designated spot in a closet. The point is, keep it all together and organized so it's less stressful to get things ready when people come over.

Another storage spot for us is under the stairs. We built a hidden door to use that typically wasted space, and that's where we keep our suitcases. We travel a lot as a family, and it's convenient to have these within reach and all in one place.

We also built a pool house that has a bathroom and a storage closet for outdoor needs, since that's a huge part of our family life. We basically live by the pool from May until September since it's so hot in Redding. In our pool storage, we keep goggles, sunscreen, pool toys, bug repellent, candles, and a medical kit (because someone's always needing a bandage!).

For a long time we had a storage unit where we stored our holiday decorations (and a million other things we didn't want in our house all year long but wanted to keep) in large, labeled containers. For those who need extra space, I highly recommended doing this. It's worth the money to have all your stuff you want to keep but don't need daily in storage. We built a barn last year, and now we store all those things in our barn.

Other People's Stuff

As you purge, you will undoubtedly find items that belong to other people. We constantly have random items left at our house, so I take a picture of each item and text it to the owner. I tell them, "I'm putting it on my porch today. Can you get it in the next few days?" If they don't pick it up or I don't know who it belongs to, it goes in the Goodwill pile. No one has time to deal with having other people's random stuff throughout their house. It adds up quickly and takes up emotional space. If you deal with things on a daily or weekly basis, you'll avoid the quicksand of procrastination to help you live more peacefully.

———

Once you go through your house room by room and purge and organize everything, you will realize how much space you were missing out on. It's a long trial-and-error process and it takes work to figure out what works best for you and your family, but it is worth it.

Looking back on the condition of my house when I first saw it, and the way it looks today, I can't help but think of all that God has done in my heart and life since then. Just like our homes, God likes to purge, organize, and renovate our hearts. And sometimes, like our homes, it takes a looooong time. But we can always trust His process. Bring God into every area of your life, the good and the mess, and follow His direction. You'll never regret it.

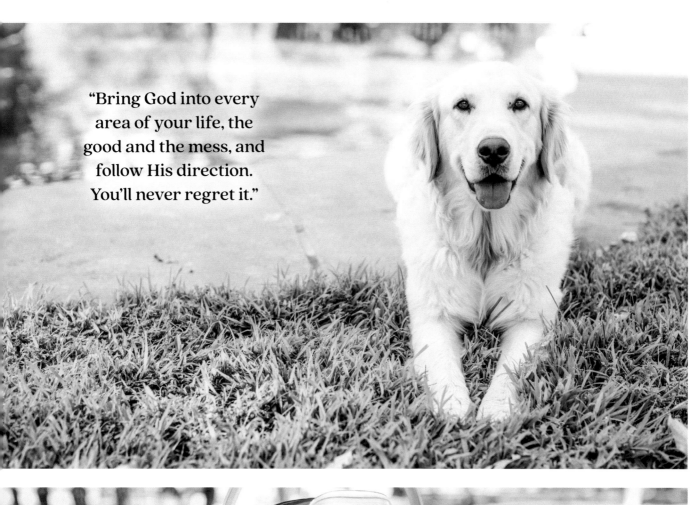

"Bring God into every area of your life, the good and the mess, and follow His direction. You'll never regret it."

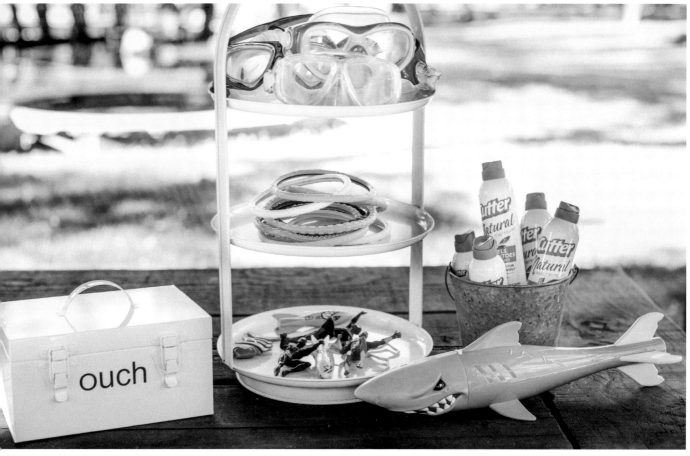

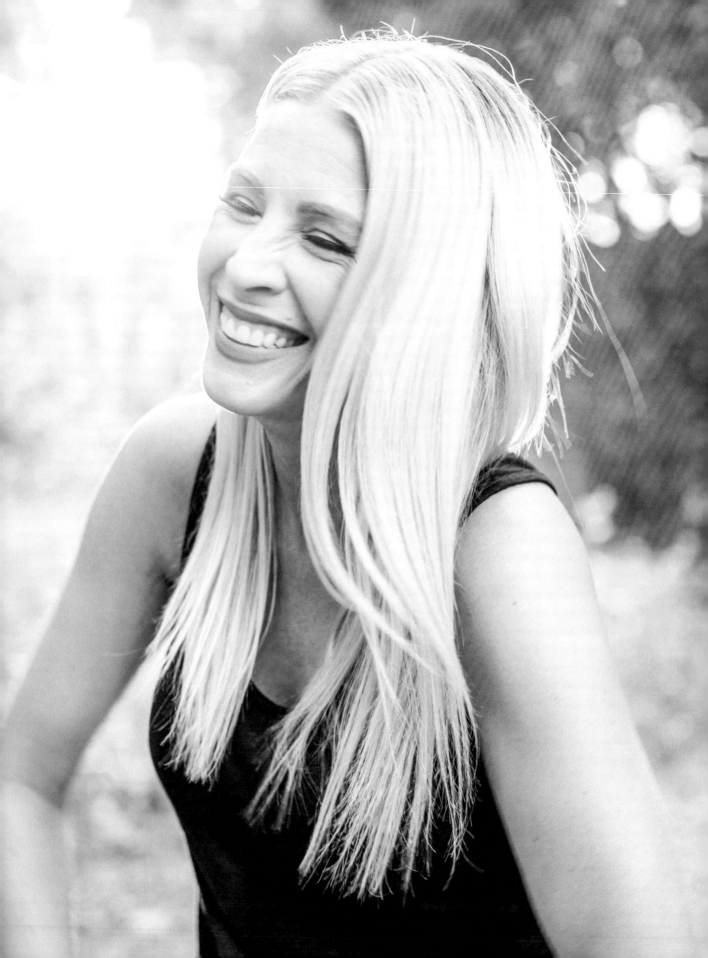

Part 02 | HEART

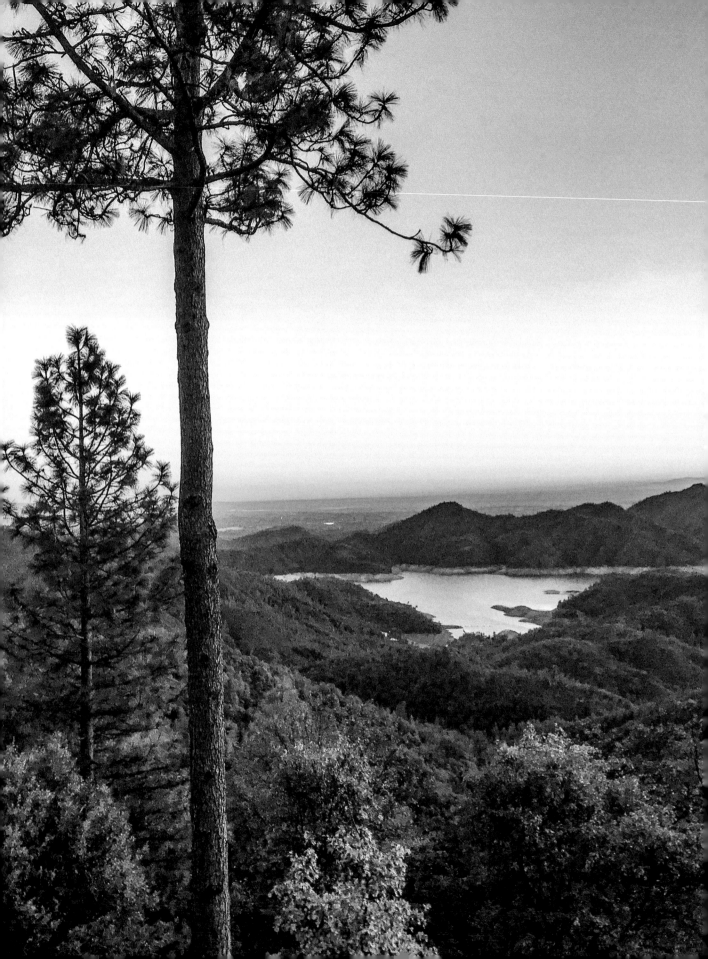

Ch. 04 | LAY IT ALL DOWN

A few years ago, I was sitting outside a friend's cabin at the top of a mountain that overlooks Redding, the town in Northern California where we live.

I was completely overwhelmed with life, trying to do *all the things*—like so many of us attempt to do, right? We were in the midst of our intense, nine-year house rebuild, and on top of that we were running Bethel Music with our friend Joel, leading worship and worship teams at our local church, touring, writing, recording, pastoring, and more. It was a lot. It was a mix of worship, community, suitcases, sawdust, pacifiers, and not much sleep. It was wild and wonderful . . . but also very overwhelming.

As I sat up there on the mountain, everything felt swirly and chaotic. I was thankful for everything we had been given and all that God was doing, but it was difficult to manage it all. My heart was heavy and I needed wisdom and clarity. **I needed to hear God speak to me.** He always brings order to chaos, shows me what to let go of and how to prioritize. **He makes it simple.** (It's one of the million reasons why I love Him.) I asked the Holy Spirit to show me where God was leading me—and where He wasn't. I took a long, honest inventory of my life at the moment. All the good stuff. All the junk. All the dreams and all the things I needed to work on.

In a way, it was like putting my life on the table—not holding anything back—and asking God to go through it with me. The Bible says, "Search me, God, and know my heart; test me and know my anxious thoughts. See if there is any offensive way in me, and lead me in the way everlasting" (Ps. 139:23–24). I needed God to show me what to keep (like my husband and the kids, duh!); what to do less (like weeding out some social obligations and projects); and what to get rid of (like the need to control and unforgiveness). I needed Him to help me go through the junk that had accumulated in my heart. As we sat together over that metaphorical table, I asked God to be really clear with me and lead my heart in the right direction. I closed my eyes, surrendered my whole life yet again, and waited for God to speak to my heart.

And then . . . He did just that.

It was like in the *Mary Poppins* scene when Mary's standing in the middle of the bedroom, snapping her fingers, and everything starts to go where it belongs. God did just that with the things taking up space in my heart, mind, and spirit. The cloudiness lifted as God put all the things exactly where they should be. (Even purging a few.)

God loves freedom, but He also loves structure and order. He loves growth, but He also loves to prune. He showed me what to focus on and what to set aside in that season. I chose to let go of what He *wasn't* highlighting and focus on what He was.

That day was a clear reminder that I need to frequently check in with God and ask Him to search my heart. He wants to lead me in what should stay and what should go in every new season. I wrote the song "I Can Feel You" (with the help of some friends) coming out of that encounter with God. That song is so special to me because it marks the beginning of a transformation in my life and a deeper connection to God as He pruned away the things that were overwhelming me and keeping me from walking in the peace He had for me. My heart for this song was that it would help people realize how close God is to us, that taking time to sit in His presence brings clarity, hope, and courage, and that we are anchored in Him no matter what life throws at us.

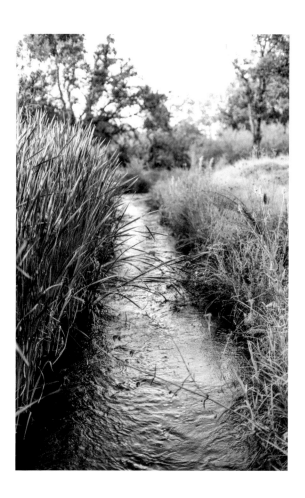

I Can Feel You—

The wind and waves surround me
I'm tossed, feel like I'm drowning
I am tired, I am weak
I need You here with me
'Cause I can feel the rising tide
But I don't have the strength to fight
I feel clouded and confused
I need You here with me
In the chaos of the storm
I have drifted far, far away
But I call out Your name
And You are just a breath
A breath away
Then through the shadows
Your light appears
I've known You're with me
But now it is clear
I can feel You,
Jesus, all around
Like sun on my skin
Warm to the touch
Here You surround me
I am held by love
I can feel You,
Jesus, all around
Now hope is rushing through my veins
'Cause everything You've rearranged
I am peaceful; I am brave
When You're here with me
All my questions find their answers here
When You come You change the atmosphere
I am focused; I am clear
When You're here with me
There is nothing in this world
That can satisfy my soul like You do
Through the storm it rages
I won't be moved
I won't be shaken
I'm anchored in You
I can feel You,
Jesus all around.

(2013)

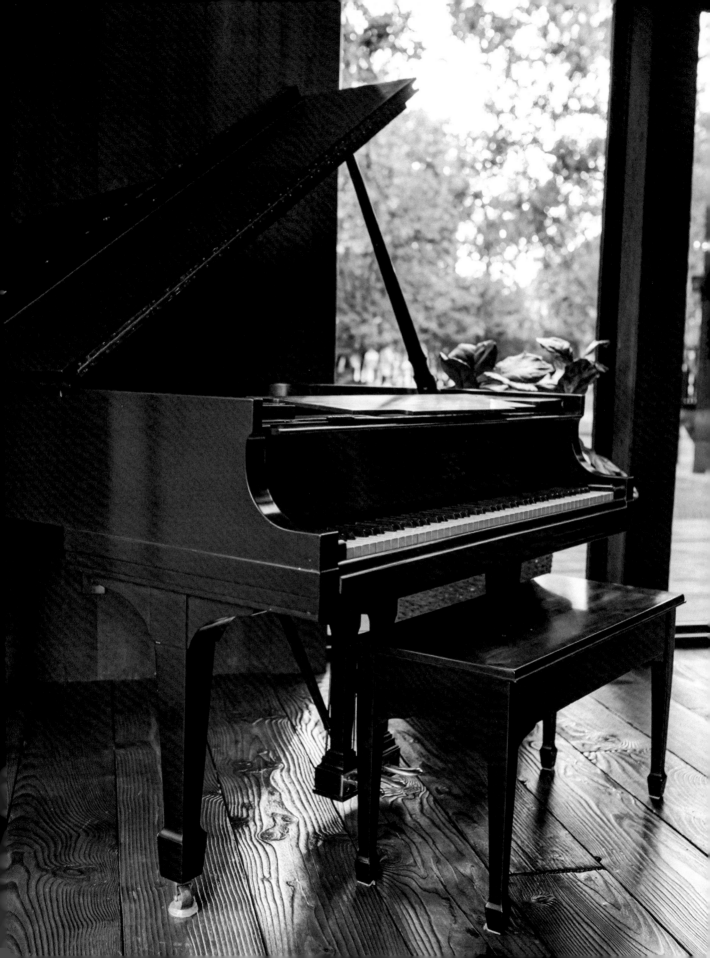

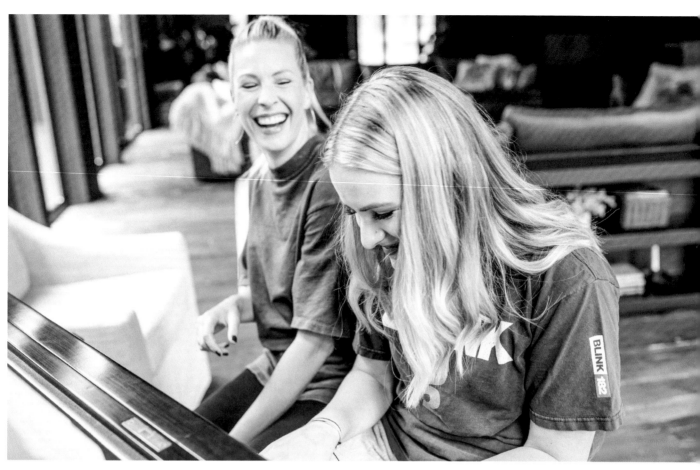

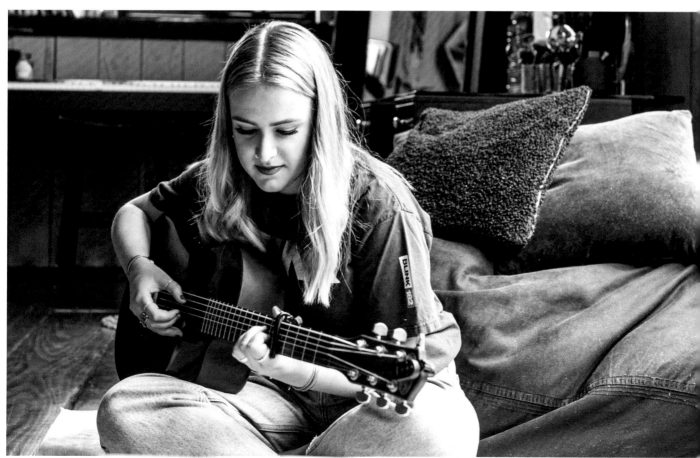

> "When we recognize the emotional junk taking up space in our hearts, we are better able to walk in purity, find healing, and worship freely."

I drove home from the mountain that day and started to make big changes to things that were draining me and our family. I talked to Brian and we rolled up our sleeves and started changing things to get our house, calendar, and, well . . . our lives into this "new order." We worked on our health, date nights, parenting, teams, house, friendships, social media purging, and much more. We knew it would be a huge renovation—just like the house rebuild we were in the middle of—but we knew we could do it. God had given us clarity, and we trusted Him completely.

We followed the direction God had shown us, and as the months passed, we really started to feel the peace in our family. We did inner healing sessions and counseling—facing things head-on and releasing bitterness, anger, and control. We still make mistakes and have to clean them up and there is a lot we are both working on, but God is gracious and kind. He guides, helps, and teaches us as we grow. I think our desire to grow and knowing that we need to grow is half the battle. Maybe that's one of the reasons God started the whole Bible with a garden: Eden, a visual of God walking with us as He tends and grows us, like a gardener.

I love that David asks God in Psalm 139 to search his heart, because it signifies humility. God knows him better than he knows himself—He is able to see beyond what David recognizes. Sometimes we know when the junk is there in our hearts; sometimes we have no idea. **We bury our pain, hang on to anger, or push back the feelings we never expressed or had the ability to release.** This is the kind of junk that isn't always obvious on the surface of our lives—we can get really good at stuffing it down or just ignoring it—but it needs to come out and be dealt with in a healthy way instead of letting it build up until it causes a breakdown. This is why asking God to search our hearts is essential.

One way or another, the junk drawer of your heart will seep into your daily life. Maybe you don't understand why you feel "blocked," maybe it reveals itself in the way you pull back from community and close relationships. Maybe it shows up in the way you never stop to rest or the way you avoid any sort of conflict. **Often, when we've done a good job of suppressing our worries or feelings, we don't even realize doing so is contributing to weighing down our hearts. But that's where the Holy Spirit can help.**

Just like that day on the mountaintop when God helped me lay everything out on the table, we need Him to walk us through an inventory of what's going on in our hearts and purge whatever is keeping us from connecting with others and God. When I am taking inventory of my heart, I ask the Holy Spirit to reveal any impurity, unresolved pain, and unforgiveness. When we recognize the emotional junk taking up space in our hearts, we are better able to walk in purity, find healing, and worship freely.

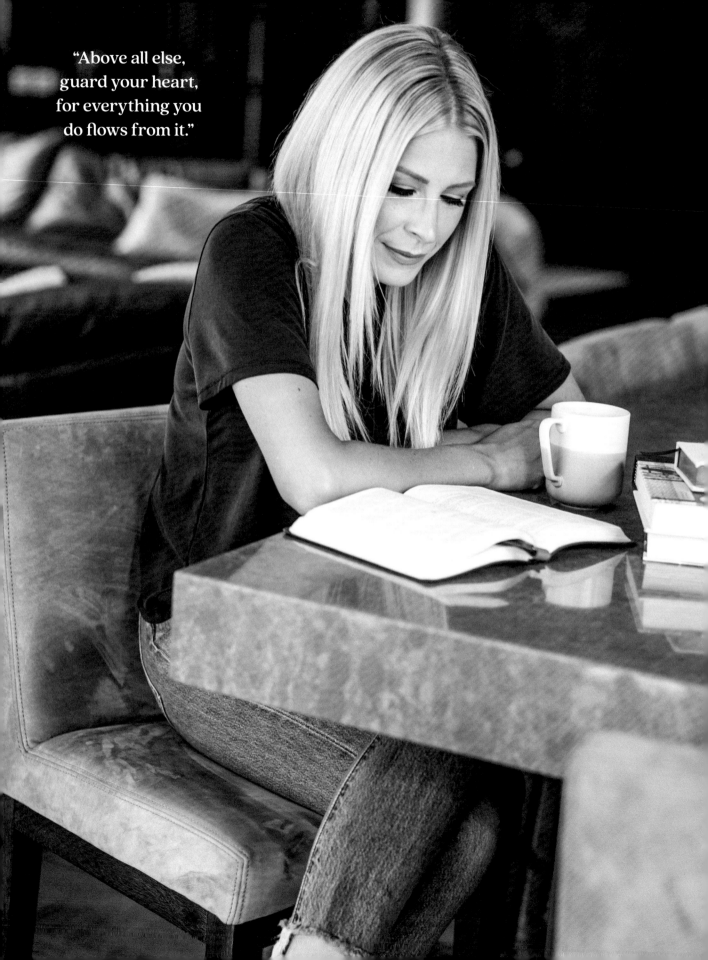

"Above all else,
guard your heart,
for everything you
do flows from it."

Ch. 05 | CLARITY AND PURITY

Keeping your life pure isn't a popular topic. We don't really want to be challenged on things that seem small or insignificant, like the Netflix series we're obsessed with or the stuff we're looking at on our phones every day.

But this is how I think about it: When you've got a dryer full of clothes that you worked hard to gather, load, and wash . . . but then you throw in something nasty (like dog poop), everything in that dryer becomes affected—not just parts of it. The same thing happens when you're following God and doing what you can to bring truth, purity, goodness, and all things lovely into your life (like reading your Bible, following His Spirit, worshipping, avoiding evil, working to be emotionally healthy, etc.), but then you consume a bunch of unhealthy junk. It seeps into your heart, your belief system, and even your dreams at night. And the same goes for food . . . just because you take vitamins and eat vegetables does not make chemical-filled nacho cheese good for you. (Oh, how I wish it was good for me, because I *love* that stuff.) The goal is to have everything in your life match the direction of where you're going so that you become a healthier, wholehearted person.

I think the most practical advice is to turn your focus onto things that are true, noble, right, pure, lovely, admirable, excellent, and praiseworthy (see Phil. 4:8); and "above all else, guard your heart, for everything you do flows from it" (Prov. 4:23).

What we consume and meditate on affects us whether we want it to or not; it's as simple as that.

If I watch a show with a lot of profanity in it, the next time I'm frustrated, profanity is instantly right there in my brain and sometimes comes right out. We can kid ourselves and say things don't affect us . . . but they do. We are called to keep our hearts pure and in order, not letting anything and everything in. And the same goes for media/social media.

Our life in Jesus is not "go-with-the-flow." We are called to be **intentional** with everything we do! **The details matter. We need to carefully consider what we're watching and listening to.** When we **avoid careless consumption,** it is easier to be consumed by what is true, honorable, right, pure, lovely, and admirable.

 pro TIP Don't walk blindly into watching something! Read about what's in a show or movie before you watch it. Be aware. If something convicts you when you're reading the description, skip it. You won't regret it. And avoid the explore page on social media . . . don't get distracted and fall into the quicksand of sin.

WATCH WHAT YOU WATCH

When I was younger, a show came out that everyone and their mom was obsessed with. The basis of the show was a group of friends with no moral compass who were sleeping around and hanging out at a coffee shop. (You know the one.) I wanted to watch it so badly! But I *knew* I wasn't supposed to watch it. Not because of my parents' rules, but because I had asked the Holy Spirit to lead every aspect of my life . . . and I knew He was telling me not to watch it because the show wouldn't be good for me. Looking back on it, I know that decision to not watch it positively affected me and saved me from a lot of emotional junk.

When we keep our lives set apart from the stuff that goes against His perfect way, we are healthier and happier. Just like Adam and Eve in the Garden of Eden with the tree they weren't supposed to eat from, He wants us to avoid what's not good for us so we can be emotionally, spiritually, and physically (holistically) healthy!

If you're a parent (or leader), other than keeping what you're consuming in check, you also have another role: helping your kids or team to navigate the same. One of the best things we've found to aid in this is keeping communication open. Checking in: asking how they're doing with friends, social media, tough situations, or anything else the Holy Spirit brings to mind to ask them. Another thing we do for our older kids is when they ask to watch a certain movie, we tell them to check out the IMDb parental guidance description, then they tell *us* if it looks like something they should be watching. It's a good training ground and it gets them into the habit of considering beforehand. Otherwise, it's just so easy to slip into careless consumption of trash.

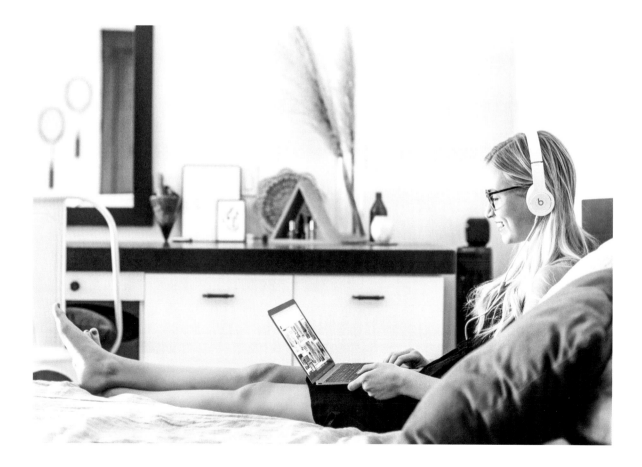

It can be hard to live counterculturally, to not be consumed by what is trending in the world, but the Bible makes it clear that is exactly what is needed:

> Don't set the affections of your heart on this world or in loving the things of the world. The love of the Father and the love of the world are incompatible. For all that the world can offer us—the gratification of our flesh, the allurement of the things of the world, and the obsession with status and importance—none of these things come from the Father but from the world. This world and its desires are in the process of passing away, but those who love to do the will of God live forever.

1 John 2:15–17 TPT

So, "watch what you watch." Keep your focus on things that please God and, more importantly, don't break God's heart, and you will experience more joy and peace. For example, as a wife, I never want to do anything that would break my husband's heart. Because I love and cherish him and my desire for purity and holiness flows from that.

I love how this verse puts it: "Let us throw off everything that hinders and the sin that so easily entangles" (Heb. 12:1). When we know God's heart for us, we don't want anything that's not holy to seep into our lives. We'll actually start seeing trash (sin and everything that entangles us) for what it is: a false fix for human desire, instant gratification, and a substitute for love! First Corinthians 6:18 clearly lays out how to live in a way that glorifies God: "Run from sexual sin!" (NLT). (This includes even the subtle stuff.)

"One of the best things we've found to aid in keeping consumption in check is keeping communication open."

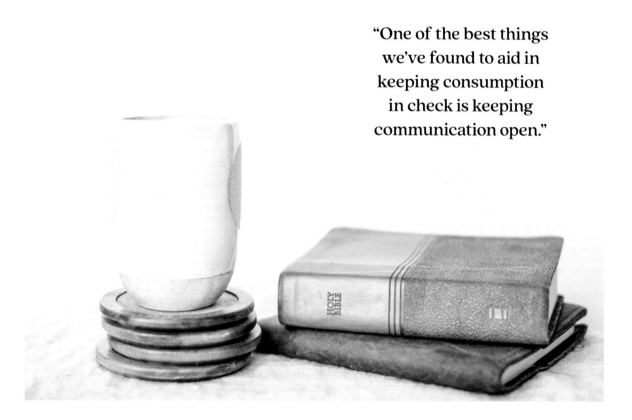

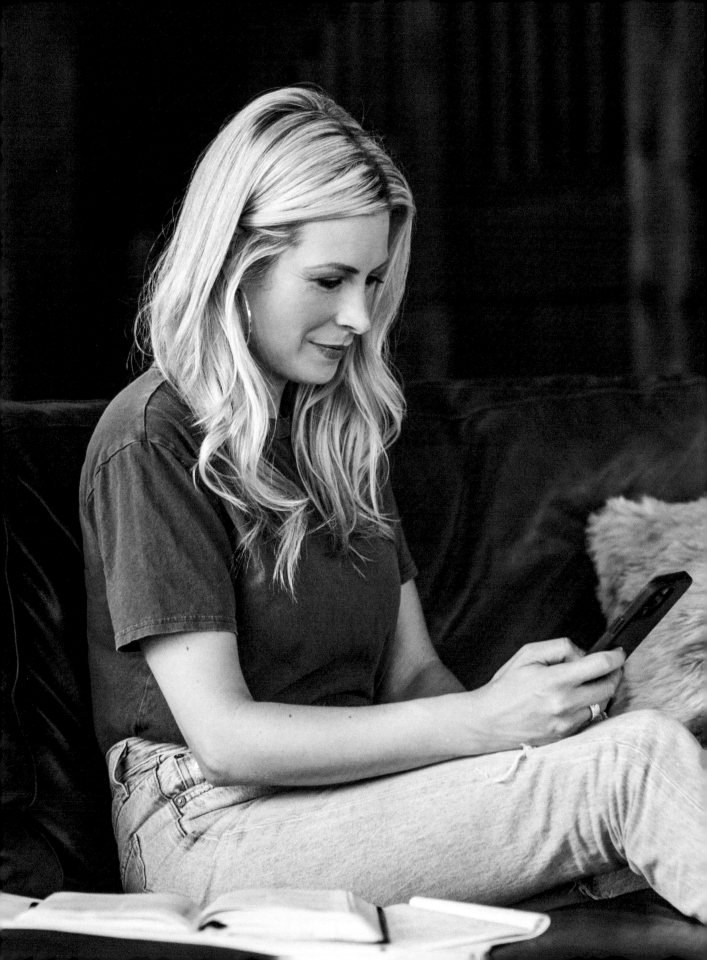

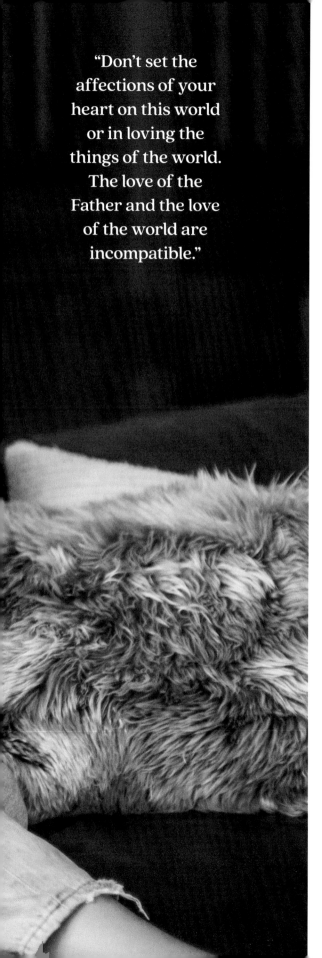

> "Don't set the affections of your heart on this world or in loving the things of the world. The love of the Father and the love of the world are incompatible."

As you're intentional about avoiding the junk, you'll notice some of the junk is obvious—like the movie that you know has trash in it or the person who posts inappropriate stuff on social media. But it's also really important to **pay attention to what alters your heart and emotions**. It could be depressing music, topics that trigger unstable emotional places, podcasts that fill you with aggression, or magazines that turn you toward envy.

Don't ignore conviction.

Ask yourself some simple questions:

1 | Would Jesus be proud of everything in this?

2 | Does everything in this represent how Jesus wants me to live?

3 | What needs of mine is this meeting in an unhealthy way?

4 | Why do I want to watch this?

WHO YOU FOLLOW

I have a love-hate relationship with social media. It's an amazing tool for getting God's word and kingdom message into the world, connecting people and spreading good, but it's also a fast track for everything unhealthy: lust, envy, pride, anger, division, lies, and all things inappropriate. Clearly, it's a mixed bag.

A couple of years ago, I was at the place of either deleting social media or following only ten people. Feeling heavy as I scrolled through, I heard God kindly say to me, *Time to unfollow anyone I tell you to.* So, I opened Instagram to the list of people I follow, and I just started going down the list of names, asking the Holy Spirit to highlight the ones to unfollow. Some of the "unfollows" made sense to me, but some were surprising. I decided to live on the safe side. Even if I didn't understand *why* it was

Clarity and Purity

> ## "It's always better to lay down your right to understand, and just obey. Again, always trusting that He knows best for your life."

good for me to unfollow a person right then, I've learned that it's always better to lay down your right to understand, and just obey. Again, always trusting that He knows best for your life.

I ended up unfollowing about two hundred people that day, and I felt the relief and peace that come when you do something you know is good for you. I did upset a few of the people I unfollowed, but when they asked me about it, I told them I was sorry, I still loved them . . . but I was trying to follow the Holy Spirit even when I didn't understand the "why." The truth is, our hearts have only so much capacity to care about things. Just like there is finite space in our homes, there is finite space in our hearts. We aren't God. Sometimes, it's simply about capacity!

Even if we follow only "healthy Christians," the highs and lows of their lives being constantly in front of us can cause our minds and emotions to be thrown around like crazy. Highs and lows, for hours a day, from so many lives will distract us and interfere with other things we're meant to be doing. More often than not, all the social media chaos ends up taking us to places that aren't emotionally healthy anyway—like jealousy, anger, depression, and confusion. Often I find myself waking up happy, and then the moment I start to scroll, depending on what's posted or going on in the world, I all of a sudden have boxing gloves on and I'm in reaction mode about something. I don't ever want to live in reaction. Response, yes, but never forced reaction.

There's much injustice in the world and many things to be passionate about and fight for, but we can't fight for everything. No one was meant to live like that . . . constantly fighting. For example, my friend Christine Caine runs a global organization that is fighting human trafficking. I am passionate about that and I support her, but I don't fight for that in the way she does. I fight what and how I'm called to, like

trying to smooth out the emotional roller coaster of the adoption process (court, birth moms, paperwork, evaluations, waiting). Different battle; same war. The point is, we have a capacity and a "lane" in which to fight, and maybe you need to find your God-given lane to make sure you're not taking on someone else's. Otherwise, you'll exhaust yourself and you'll be kept from the area in which God wants you to fight.

Social media can quickly distract me from priorities in my life. I have watched it deplete me of the emotional capacity I require for the people who are physically in my day-to-day life and who need me. When that happens, it's time for some parameters—like going on social media only at a certain time in the day . . . not throughout the day. Or if you know social media is taking you to unhealthy places, just *let it go*. Delete it from your phone. Unfollow a ton of people. But the point is . . . **guard your heart.** You will find whole new levels of clarity and be able to invest your time in what and who you're called to!

Matthew 6:22 tells us, "The eye is the lamp of the body. If your eyes are healthy, your whole body will be full of light." Imagine how good it would feel to have your whole body be full of light. *That* would be true freedom. No shame. No regret. Again, don't be overwhelmed . . . God's got you, and He will lead you every step of the way. Simply ask Him to help you hear His voice and increase your sensitivity. He'll do it.

BE AWARE OF WHAT YOU MAGNIFY

We've talked about who you're following and what you're taking in—but let's take a minute to talk about what you put *out* into the world. What you talk about, write, sing, create, teach . . . it matters!

Jesus is calling all of us higher, to be set apart. In our family, church, record label, and worship community, we're passionate about purity and holiness. We take 1 Timothy 4:12 to heart when it says, **"Set an example for the believers in speech, in conduct, in love, in faith and in purity."** We are all leaders . . . we are *leading* people to Christ; and we are called to live "above reproach" (1 Tim. 3:2), which means we must dedicate ourselves to **live in a way in which no one can find fault**.

We all have blind spots and we need to be there to help one another see those blind spots—where we're weak and need to grow. This could look like a phone call to talk through what someone did, said, or posted if it wasn't appropriate or distracted from whatever is pure, lovely, and good (see Phil. 4:8). Is that fun to do? No. It is compared to iron sharpening iron (see Prov. 27:17), and I don't know if you've ever heard the sound of iron being sharpened, but it's . . . the worst! Shrill and like nails on a chalkboard. The point is it's uncomfortable, but Jesus is calling us to help one another. Help involves not just hugs and encouragement; help involves accountability and looking out for each other. And like Proverbs 27:6 says, "Wounds from a friend can be trusted, but an enemy multiplies kisses." We need people in our lives who love us enough not only to encourage us, but also to call us out on the things we need to work on.

When you need to talk to someone about something intense . . . do so in person. Avoid communicating your message with a text or online. One of my favorite verses on this is 2 John 1:12 where Paul is writing to the churches and he says, "I have much to write to you, but I do not want to use paper and ink. Instead, I hope to visit you and talk with you face to face, so that our joy may be complete." What he's saying in our day and age is something like this: "Let's not text, email, or even talk on the phone about this. Let's talk in person." Let them feel your love. Don't let the enemy steal something through miscommunication. In a world of technology like we have (texts, emails, social media, etc.), face-to-face interaction is rare, sometimes even among friends. Nothing replaces being together, in person. It's like "online church"; it's great, but *nothing* replaces being in the room with the presence of God and His people. There's nothing like it.

Brave communication and tough conversations are a part of growth and health. Maybe you suspect that someone is doing something shady. Instead of accusing, try asking them a question about it. When we are angry, hurt, or frustrated, love can be the first thing to fly out the window. But love believes the best in people.

The Bible says this about love in the book of 1 Corinthians:

> **It does not rejoice at injustice, but rejoices with the truth [when right and truth prevail]. Love bears all things [regardless of what comes], believes all things [looking for the best in each one], hopes all things [remaining steadfast during difficult times], endures all things [without weakening]. Love never fails.**
>
> *13:6–8 AMP*

Proverbs 18:21 says, "Your words are so powerful that they will kill or give life, and the talkative person will reap the consequences" (TPT). We've all seen this play out! We know how it feels to be torn apart by someone's words, or emotionally triggered, or thrown off our course. But we also know how it feels to experience the opposite: words that bring light and hope, encourage us, make us better people, challenge us, and help us "press toward the mark for the prize of the high calling of God in Christ Jesus" (Phil. 3:14 KJV).

"Your words are so powerful that they will kill or give life, and the talkative person will reap the consequences."

Clarity and Purity

Most importantly, does what you're saying, posting, and putting out into the world magnify God? Does it magnify the good that is happening? Yes, there's evil in the world—but why magnify it when we know God overcomes all darkness? My Bible says, "Oh, magnify the LORD with me, and let us exalt his name together!" (Ps. 34:3 ESV). We must be people who go higher and bring light to the darkness by displaying and magnifying the good instead. Want to magnify justice? Magnify how someone is doing it right versus how someone is doing it wrong. Want to magnify truth? Speak and amplify truth rather than just pointing out lies and falsehoods. Study and reflect what is *real, true, and good* and lead others in the same direction. This doesn't mean we never talk or post about difficult things, but we have to watch what we magnify.

My father-in-law, Bill, has a great quote: "If God inhabits my praise, who inhabits my complaints?" Whether it's social media, TV shows, what you're listening to or reading, evaluate all the things you're consuming. What's taking up valuable space without offering you good? What's causing you emotional chaos? Does it line up with who you want to be? Guard your heart and . . .

Don't let evil conquer you, but conquer evil by doing good.

Romans 12:21 NLT

To be clear: This is *not* about judgment or creating shame. This is about looking stuff directly in the face, getting really honest, and letting the Holy Spirit help us clear out our lives so He can lead us to health and joy.

Pause and consider:

- For social media purging, open your account and run down the list of the people you follow. Ask the Holy Spirit to give you a check on any people or accounts you should unfollow, and then unfollow them. (I highly recommend following only people who lead you toward Jesus.)

- Just like assessing the people you're following, ask yourself, *Why are people following me? Am I leading them to Jesus and His Word, family, healing, the beauty of the church, worship, encouragement, and positivity . . . or just constant selfies, opinions, church hate, negativity, people shaming, and self-promotion?* We have to remember why we are on this planet—and it's not just to post random things. We have a responsibility with *all* that we've been given (including our social media) to show God and His kingdom to the world. If you need to make adjustments or delete some things right now, do it. Walk a new path.

- For news and current events, take a minute to consider how much time and energy you spend consuming news and opinions. What's it doing for your heart and emotions? Are you getting sidetracked by others' offenses? Would you experience more peace if you pulled back?

- Think about specific topics that send you down an emotional, confused, or unhealthy path. What seems to pull you in, but then leaves you feeling terrible afterward?

To stay healthy, you'll need to constantly assess your physical and emotional world with the Holy Spirit and, just like in any garden, let Him pull the weeds out. Because for anything to grow best, weeds have to be removed frequently.

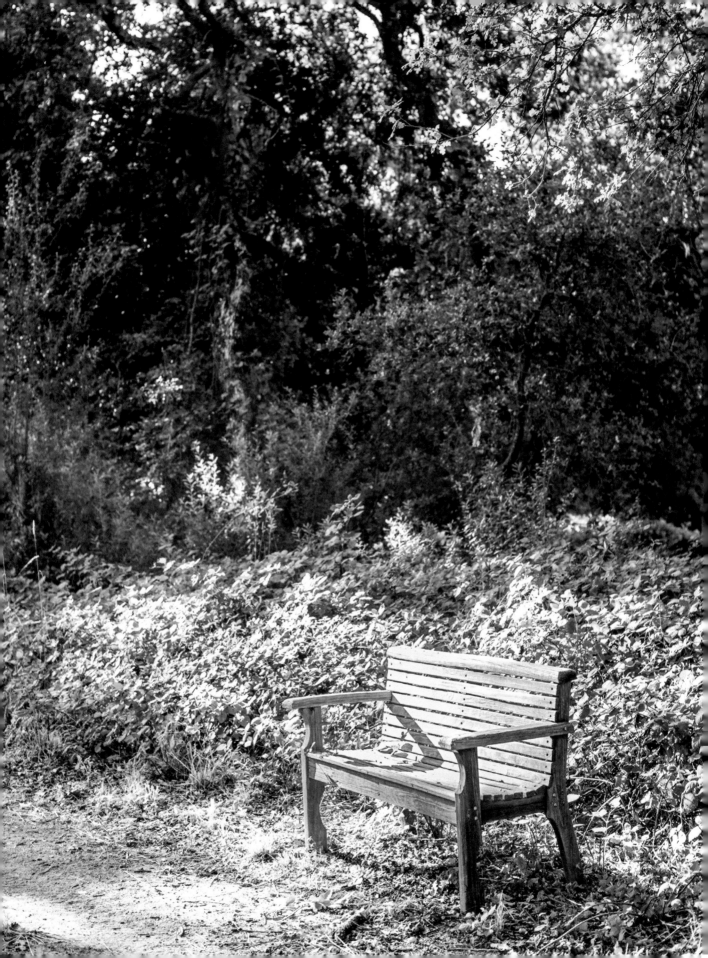

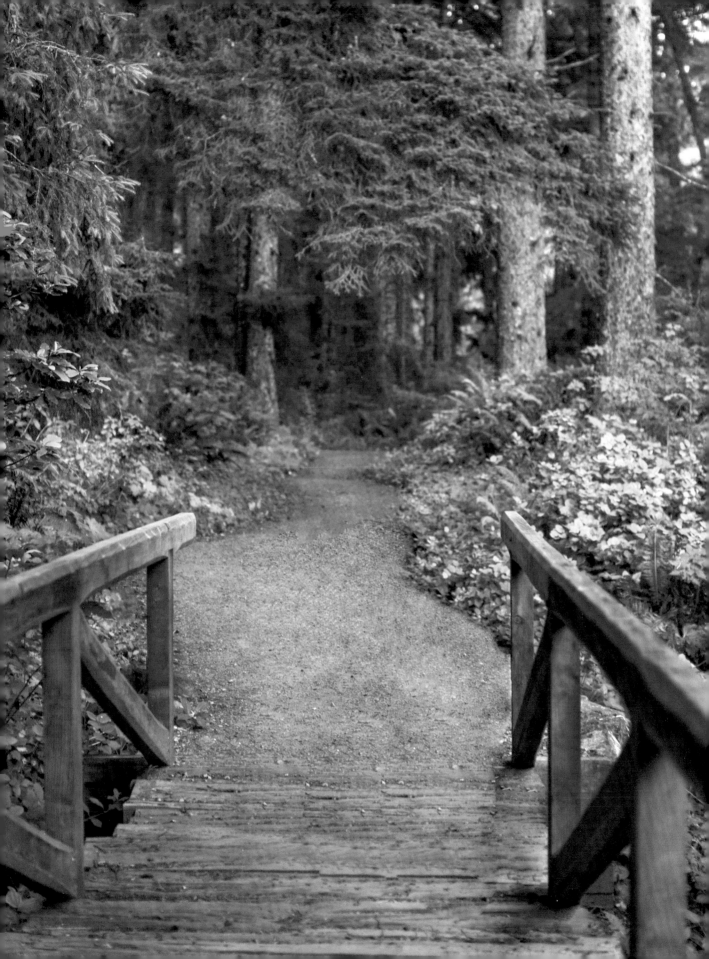

HEALING

We can set boundaries and guard our hearts against the temptations and things of this world to the best of our ability (see Prov. 4:23; 1 John 2:15), but sometimes junk gets into our hearts unintentionally.

I call it being "slimed" (this goes back to my being a child of the '80s and my love for the TV show *Double Dare*). The emotional junk builds up if we don't deal with it and causes disorder and confusion in our lives.

A few years ago, my husband had a nervous breakdown. I still remember every moment so clearly—the afternoon it happened, the months he was like a medicated vegetable in our home, and, thankfully, the breakthrough and freedom that finally came. As Brian healed, he wrote an incredible book (*When God Becomes Real*), in which he tells the story of what happened and how he got through it. I want to tell you some of that story here too. Because I believe that if we're going to "get our houses in order," our hearts need close attention as well. And it's often in hearing **the testimonies of others** that **you will find healing**. As Revelation tells us, "**They overcame him by the blood of the Lamb, and by the word of their testimony**" (12:11 KJV).

When Brian went to the doctor after the breakdown, he told him about the stress and pressure that had been building. The doctor nodded along and said, "Your body might be showing you your limits. There is only so much stress and tension you can fill your body with. There comes a point where the brain can't handle any more, and everything just sort of shuts down."

Brian writes in *When God Becomes Real*:

[The doctor] exposed a truth hidden in plain sight. I'd been so busy that I hadn't stopped to consider the combined weight of the stress, pressure and conflict. And even if I did, it wasn't anything I could just quit . . . But the things we were involved in weren't the problem. Over the years, I'd taken the negative emotion, every frustration and hurt, and I'd pushed it down, thinking if I ignored it, it would all go away. It didn't. All those emotions that I had not dealt with finally caught up with me.

The next months of our lives were filled with an entirely new reality. Medication to fight the intense panic attacks, counseling sessions, scary lows, hour upon hour of worship, and wondering if he'd ever win the mental fight and get to a place of peace . . . or back to normal. The weight and responsibility of taking care of him, the house, kids, and work were on my shoulders for the most part. He was medicated to

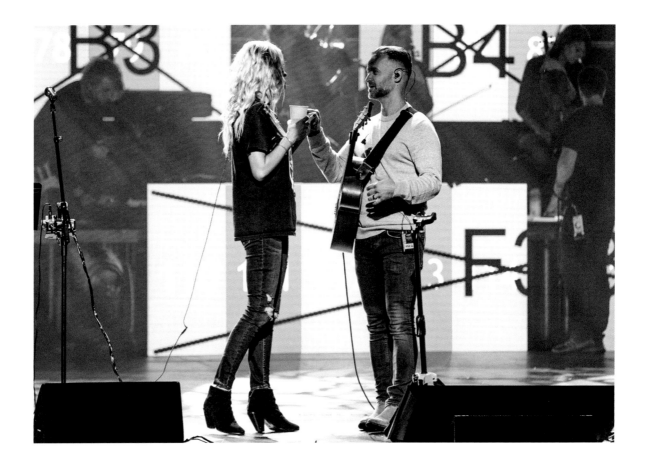

keep his mind calm, and I definitely battled thoughts of *Will this be how he is from now on?*

After a few months, I had come to the end of my rope. I was exhausted. I remember lying on my bed, tears streaming down my face, and talking to God. A verse popped into my mind: *Lamentations 3:28*. I had no idea what that verse said, so I grabbed my Bible next to the bed and looked it up. I love the way Eugene Peterson phrases that passage in *The Message* translation:

> When life is heavy and hard to take, go off by yourself. Enter the silence. Bow in prayer. Don't ask questions: Wait for hope to appear. Don't run from trouble. Take it full-face. The "worst" is never the worst.
>
> *Lamentations 3:28–30, emphasis added*

Those words jumped off the page. I heard God speak to me: *This isn't the worst. It will get better.* And even though each day after that wasn't easy by any means, I knew God was with me and it wouldn't last forever. It was in that season I wrote the song "You're Gonna Be OK." It became an anchor for me—a prophetic promise for Brian and our family.

> "Those words jumped off the page. I heard God speak to me: *This isn't the worst. It will get better.*"

You're Gonna Be OK

———————————

I know it's all you've got to just be strong
And it's a fight just to keep it together, together
I know you think that you are too far gone
But hope is never lost, hope is never lost

Hold on, don't let go
Hold on, don't let go
Just take one step closer
Put one foot in front of the other
You'll get through this
Just follow the light in the darkness
You're gonna be OK

I know your heart is heavy from those nights
But just remember that you are a fighter,
a fighter
You never know just what tomorrow holds
And you're stronger than you know, stronger
than you know

Hold on, don't let go
Hold on, don't let go
Just take one step closer
Put one foot in front of the other
You'll get through this
Just follow the light in the darkness
One step closer
Put one foot in front of the other
You'll get through this
Just follow the light in the darkness
You're gonna be OK
And when the night is closing in
Don't give up and don't give in
This won't last, it's not the end, it's not the end
You're gonna be OK
When the night is closing in
Don't give up and don't give in
This won't last, it's not the end, it's not the end
You're gonna be OK

(2016)

I believed Brian would be okay. I believed God would heal him. But sometimes it's a long road.

At one point in the midst of this, I thought that just getting out of town together could be a good thing for both of us, so we packed our bags, dropped the kids at Grandma's, and headed to one of our favorite places, Napa Valley. But even staying in a beautiful hotel and eating at restaurants we loved . . . it just wasn't helping. Brian's anxiety was so present, even as much as he tried to push it away and enjoy what was right in front of us. Like we'd been doing for months, he'd give me the look, his eyes wide with fear, and we'd leave the restaurant or stop what we were doing and pray through the panic episode. Many nights I'd stay awake with him, praying over him, trying to reassure him that it was going to be okay, that he wasn't losing his mind.

We left to return home from our trip early and were so disappointed with how it had gone. It wasn't the getaway we needed, and we felt like we had tried everything and nothing was changing. After about an hour into our drive, I could sense Brian's panic growing. An idea popped into my head (thanks, Jesus). I turned to him and asked, "Babe, who do you need to forgive?" He began to talk through people and things that had caused him pain in his past. I wanted to make space for everything he was feeling so it wouldn't stay bottled in. Brian thought he had fully processed the hurt and frustrations from his past, but it became clear that he hadn't. Brian recounts, "I believed in inner healing and was sure I had dealt with any areas of unforgiveness. But this moment was different. I'd been pushed into a corner, and it finally allowed me to see it all in a new light."

I knew God was doing some deep inner healing. **The Holy Spirit brought to mind the names of people that he needed to forgive.** He started naming people out loud that he felt bitterness toward. Brian wrote about this experience in *When God Becomes Real*:

> As I began to confess this bitterness, as I spoke the names out loud, I saw my own part in some of the messes. I'd made small choices, done things that had seemed inconsequential at the time. I'd failed to communicate or avoided conflict altogether. I began to see how much these things mattered. The things I'd swept under the rug were amplified and highlighted as we prayed, and I could see how God was showing me just how important they were to Him.
>
> If I was going to make it to the other side of this breakdown, I couldn't hold onto any form of unforgiveness. I confessed it all and resolved to live a different way; and in that commitment, I felt a real sense of hope. **It felt like my soul was clean.** God had used this experience to prepare my heart to encounter Him in a whole new way. (emphasis added)

From there, everything began to change. Brian had surrendered all that stuff he'd pushed into the back of his heart, and once it was out and dealt with, he could breathe again. He began **living intentionally** in the present moments, **slowing himself way down**, and **meditating on Scripture** every morning. He was able to start slowly easing off the medication and navigating life without it. Even though he would still have moments of panic, his world wasn't closing in on him like before. He learned how to lean into the pain and panic and work through it with God, dealing with the root of the matter to get back into wholeness—into restoration. I love how he put it: "It felt like my soul was clean."

It was a crushing and pressing time for Brian, but the fruit that it produced in his life was amazing and he experienced a lot of healing and freedom. For our kids, watching him battle through this season **partnered with God** (God helping him)

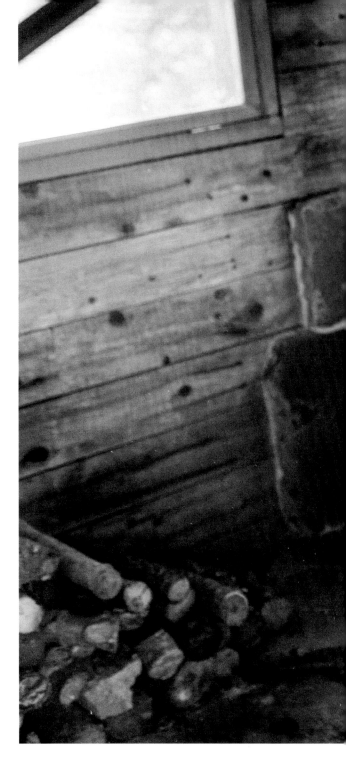

was beautiful. They watched him being crushed and pressed, but they also watched him pray and worship through it, often listening to worship music for hours on end. It really showed the kids

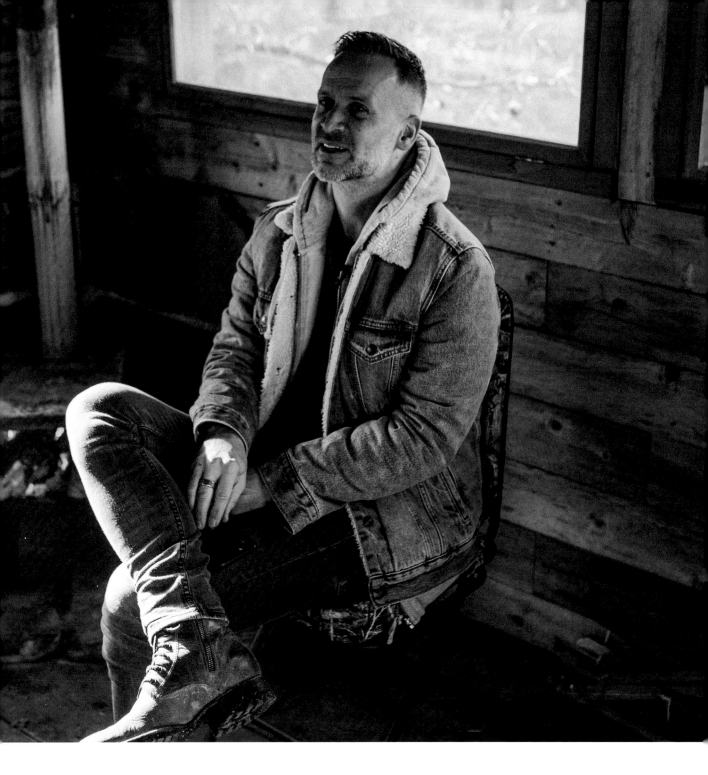

our need for God in a painful but beautiful way, and it also showed them how God is with us no matter what we go through and that He'll get us through it. Brian and I are very open with our kids, so talking with them through the whole process and even on the other side of it has been an amazing journey.

When we're working through unresolved pain, trauma, anxiety, or emotional turmoil, we have to begin making lifestyle changes that are good for our hearts and help bring healing:

1| **SEARCH YOUR HEART.** Figure out what is causing emotional buildup in your life. If there is someone you need to forgive, then forgive them. Maybe it's a long list! That's okay. Sometimes the Holy Spirit will highlight people you didn't think you even needed to forgive, but you do. Repent. Forgive.

2| **REMEMBER, WE'RE ALL HUMAN,** we all hurt people, we all need forgiveness, and we all need to forgive. We need to forgive ourselves too! Invite the Holy Spirit to show you the places of your heart that need attention and healing.

3| **HAVE THE TOUGH CONVERSATIONS.** Forgiveness and brave communication are important to God and affect our overall health and life experience. Telling people how you feel and what you need is vital. Have the tough conversations. Admit and confess. Let all that stuff come out of the shadows and into the light so you can heal and get healthy, and so you can help others do the same.

4| **LIVE INTENTIONALLY.** Find ways to stay in the present moment. Note the things that trigger you to visit dark emotional places and do your best to avoid those things. Surround yourself with people who help you get closer to Jesus, who uplift you and encourage you but who also love you enough to talk to you when you're "off."

5| **SLOW DOWN.** What is causing stress, pressure, or conflict in your life that you can cut out? What is draining you? Make a list of the things you absolutely can't cut from your life and your schedule and the things that you can. If you find yourself putting everything in the first category, let the Holy Spirit help (and maybe a Spirit-filled counselor too).

6| **MEDITATE ON SCRIPTURE.** Ask God to speak to you in His Word. Find verses and stories that relate to what you're going through. Find verses that speak to you and encourage your inner healing. God gives me a key verse for every season. Display Scripture in your car, on your desk, as your phone background. Surround yourself with it so that it fills your mind and heart.

7| **RELY ON COMMUNITY.** Our community was very supportive and helped me cope with everything going on during Brian's treatment by gathering around us to pray, encourage, and help. Being vulnerable and asking for help is hard, but we have to start opening up, letting people speak into our habits and behaviors, and asking for help when we're stuck or feeling blocked . . . whether or not we know what's causing the feeling. Even if you don't know the answer to the problem, sometimes just talking about it brings peace because you're verbalizing how you feel and what you need. Reach out and ask for prayer too! We all need it.

Healing happens when you bring things to the light. You will never heal from something you hide. If you break your arm, you don't slap a little bandage on it and move on. You get it checked out, you get surgery if needed, and then you go through the proper recovery to restore it. You can't pretend it didn't happen and move on. And sometimes a break gets worse before it gets better, right? The doctor might have to rebreak your arm to reset it. But lean into the initial mess and pain; the healing is worth it. (Similar to emptying everything out of the pantry so you can organize it.) When our souls are clean and our hearts are healed, we will have a greater capacity to do what we are on this planet to do: be like Jesus and to help others come to know Him.

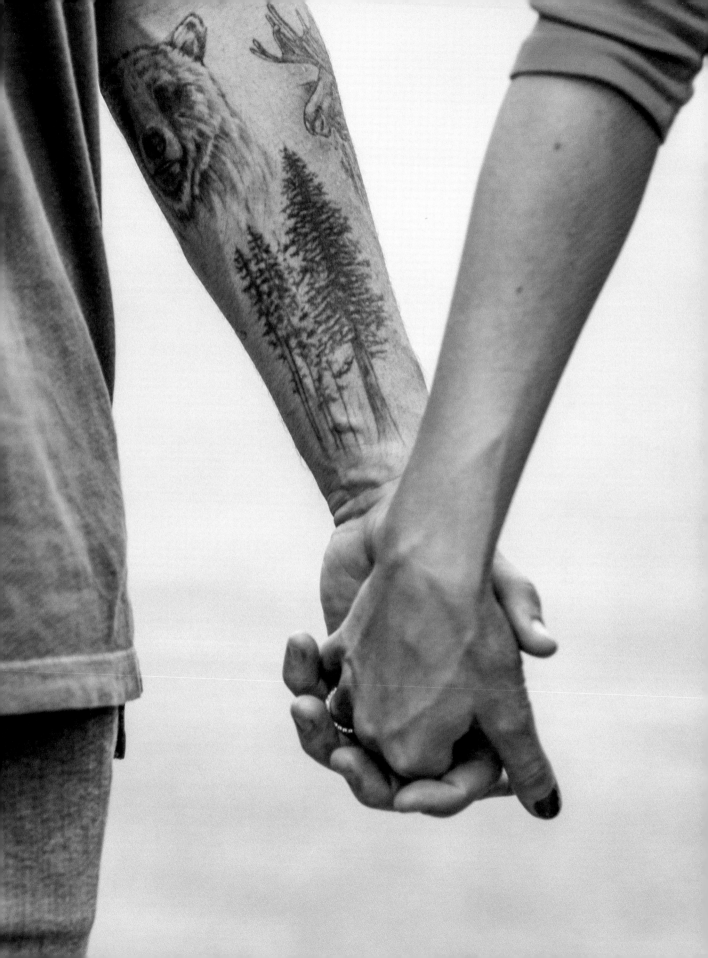

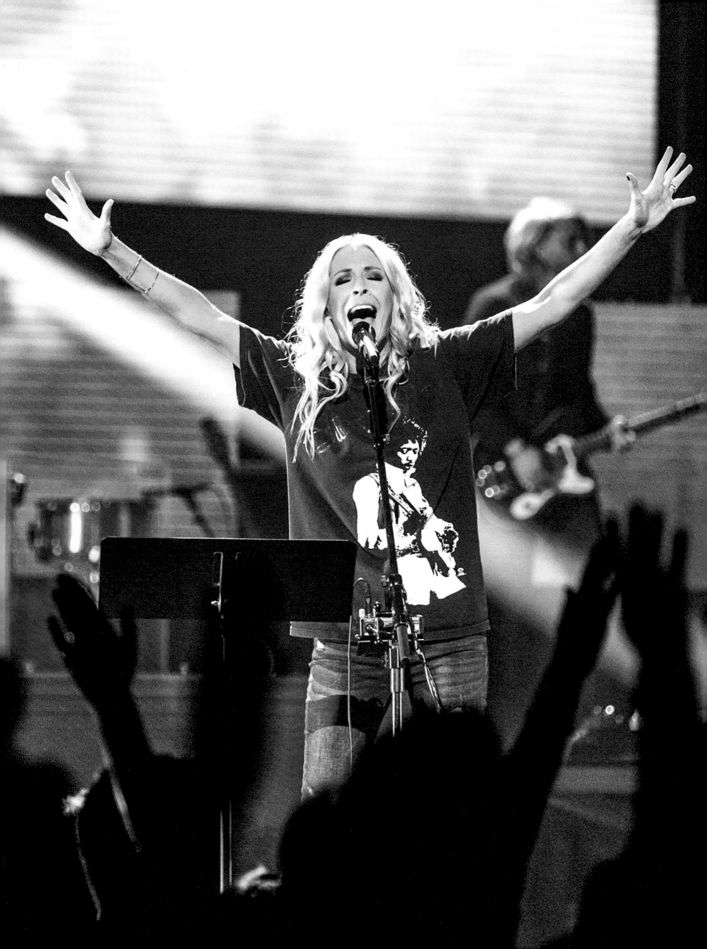

Ch. 07 | WORSHIP

I was asked one time on a panel, "Why do we worship?" I sat there a minute and then just blurted out, "How could we not?" and that's really how I feel.

God is *so* good and wonderful and close and kind, and I'm just so thankful for Him and everything He does . . . worship is a natural response to who God is.

In worship, we magnify God for who He is and celebrate who we are in and through Him. We can come before God just as we are . . . with all our emotions, the highs and lows of life, all our mess, pain, and joy . . . and our good Father is our help, our strength, and the "lifter" of our heads (see Ps. 3:3 ESV). He restores, heals, and brings hope and joy and a million other lovely things.

Worship isn't just singing or declaring; worship is your whole life, every part of it before God and for Him. Every decision, every battle, every victory . . . it's all worship. Worship is a lifestyle. Like that day on the mountain when I laid everything out before Him, my whole life, like an offering . . . that was worship. Worship is about getting our hearts right before God so we can become more like Him.

God is constantly working on my heart in worship, highlighting areas that are not in order with truth. Leading worship from a stage is a very vulnerable thing, and even if you've done it a hundred times, it can be unnerving and filled with pressure. Leading worship is all about magnifying God, hearing what He's saying in a moment and speaking or singing that, being sensitive to what He's doing in the room, all the while trying to be completely yourself. A complex combination! I remember years ago we were on tour and had just finished a worship set. It hadn't gone well in my opinion (it happens!). I walked off the stage embarrassed, feeling like I'd failed. I felt God inviting me to get away and talk to Him. I'd learned enough at that point to stop right there and then to find the space to listen. So I found a quiet spot and sat down by myself. The presence of God surrounded me.

I heard God say, *Remember who this is for and who it's about.*

I started sobbing.

Did you do your best? He asked.

"Yes," I answered.

That's all that matters.

Then God showed me a picture of a refrigerator with children's art displayed on it. He said, *It's not about perfection. It's about your heart.* When you follow the voice of God, you won't get it right one hundred percent of the time. You will look dumb sometimes as you step out in risk, but the end result is never the goal . . . Just like when I ask my kids to do a chore. It's not that they need to do it perfectly; it's their attitude, their willingness to obey, and whether they do their best that matters. When we worship and obey Him, everything in our lives comes into order.

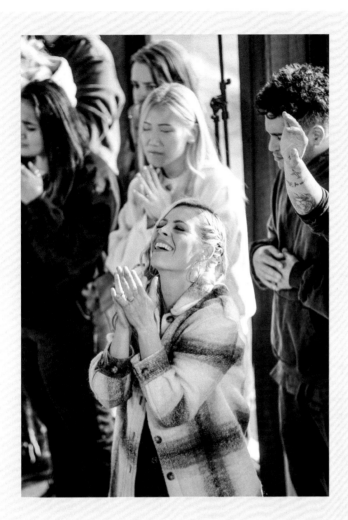

Return, O my soul, to your rest;
for the LORD has dealt bountifully
with you.
For you have delivered my soul
from death,
my eyes from tears,
my feet from stumbling.

Psalm 116:7–8 ESV

For God hath not given us the
spirit of fear; but of power, and of
love, and of a sound mind.

2 Timothy 1:7 KJV

Do not be anxious about anything,
but in everything by prayer and
supplication with thanksgiving let
your requests be made known to

I had another encounter with God once where He showed me an amazing picture of what happens when we worship. I saw us on earth praising and worshipping God, declaring that He is holy, worthy, and wonderful. Our praise and worship rose to the heavens, like incense. As it did, three things happened: First, God absorbed our worship (like when someone you love gives you a hug); second, as He absorbed the words that we were declaring, He shouted those words over the earth, declaring, "Yes, I am," in agreement. And the third thing I saw was God holding a mirror. As our praise rose to the heavens, the words ricocheted back to earth and God declared to us, His people, "So are you." Because when we worship, we become like the One we worship.

We don't worship because God is an egotist who needs to be told who He is. God is confident. We worship because, as I answered the panel question, how could we not?! God is wonderful and we worship Him for all He has done, is doing, and will do for us. Also, when we worship, we become more like Him—reflecting His image more—and that's the Father's heart for us. I love how 2 Corinthians 3:18 puts it: "And we all, who with unveiled faces **contemplate the Lord's glory, are being transformed into his image with ever-increasing glory, which comes from the Lord, who is the Spirit**" (emphasis added).

We are called to represent (and to re-present) Him.

God. And the peace of God, which surpasses all understanding, will guard your hearts and your minds in Christ Jesus.

Philippians 4:6–7 ESV

Do not be conformed to this world, but be transformed by the renewal of your mind, that by testing you may discern what is the will of God, what is good and acceptable and perfect.

Romans 12:2 ESV

If we confess our sins, he is faithful and just to forgive us our sins, and to cleanse us from all unrighteousness.

1 John 1:9 KJV

Create in me a clean heart, O God, and renew a right spirit within me.

Psalm 51:10 ESV

Set your minds on things that are above, not on things that are on earth.

Colossians 3:2 ESV

When the Spirit of truth comes, he will guide you into all truth; for he will not speak on his own authority, but whatever he hears he will speak, and he will declare to you the things that are to come.

John 16:13 RSV

I don't know about you, but for me, being in the presence of God in worship is where I feel the glory of God the strongest. And it's in those moments we are changed and made more like Him.

————

Proverbs 4:23 tells us that everything we do flows from our hearts. That means it's important to get our hearts in order! Guarding our hearts against the things of this world, opening our hearts to healing and forgiveness, having a heart for others, and worshipping in everything we do will bring health to us, our families, and our communities. Don't let any junk fill you; be filled with peace and joy so that you have more capacity for God and people.

When our hearts are right before God, we will start getting healthier in other areas of our lives as well. From our bodies, to our images, to our schedules, when we have a goal to get our "house" in order, and take small steps toward order, we will begin to experience holistic health.

————

Above are some Scriptures to give you courage and truth as you invite God to search your heart. Know that God is *for* you and He is the Healer. He wants you to experience an abundant life and not be weighed down by fear, pain, regret, mistakes, or any other negative thing. He wants to heal you and help you let go of that junk.

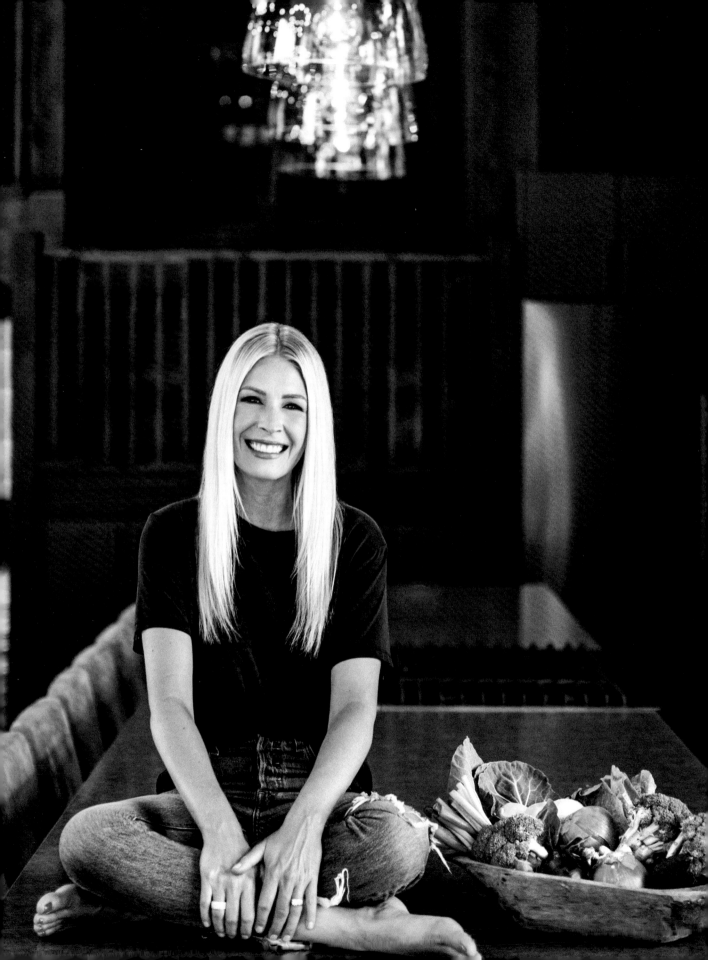

Part
03
HEALTH

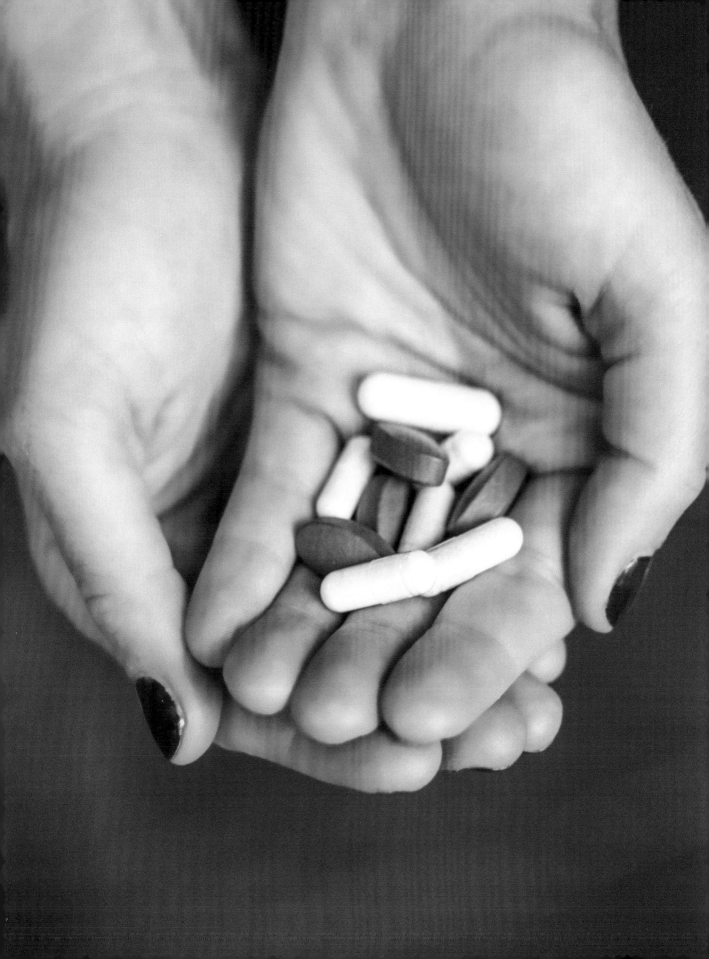

Ch. 08 | FEELING OUT OF ORDER

A few years ago, when I was thirty-five, I knew something was off in my body because I felt "out of order." I was exhausted, I felt years older than I actually was, and my body was struggling with sleep, muscle tightness, and digestion issues.

And I also had a sharp pain in my butt (literally!). I was so frustrated because I had received prayer, tried multiple physical therapists, sports massage, medications, and even injections to help with my pain, but to no avail.

At that time, I was going to weekly physical therapy, taking multivitamins, eating pretty healthy, and staying active (turns out chasing three kids around is really good exercise). And even though I could have just chalked up how I felt to the wild season of our lives we were going through, I knew something was off. I decided to dig deeper and find out what my body needed.

I went in to have my blood checked by a local doctor. She said I was a "little low in vitamins B and D" so I increased my intake of those vitamins, but her advice seemed vague, so I decided to get a second opinion. Meanwhile, my mother-in-law, who had been diagnosed with cancer, was working with a cellular biologist MD in Spain named Dr. Hilu. He had done extensive blood work on her, then treated her, and she experienced incredible results! I felt this was the next step the Holy Spirit was leading me toward, so I redid my blood work with Dr. Hilu.

When I got back the results, I couldn't believe the level of detail. Not only did Dr. Hilu say I was deficient in many vitamins and minerals, he also said I needed to be off my feet more. I rarely stopped moving except to sleep (partially because my butt hurt worse if I sat or lay down), and most of that physical movement was in short bursts cleaning around the house or chasing kids . . . not enough long-distance walking. The results of his testing totally made sense! I made three simple changes:

1 | I bought all the vitamins and minerals that my results said I needed (and I got one of those granny vitamin container systems to organize them!).

2 | I started taking intentional breaks to rest with my feet up during the day.

3 | I began taking from three- to seven-mile-long walks almost every day.

I couldn't believe how quickly my body responded. I felt twenty-five again within two weeks! My digestion issues cleared, I was sleeping better, I had energy again, and my self-esteem increased. I felt amazing—and still do. And after those three changes, the only thing left was the pain in my butt! But that story ends well here too!

Shortly after I made those adjustments, I was teaching at a medical professionals meeting about juggling work and family. Afterward, a woman came up to me and said she'd seen my online prayer request for pain relief. She told me she was a specialized physical therapist and she believed I had a piriformis problem that she could help me with. The piriformis muscle is in the buttocks (which explains my actual pain in the butt) and it can irritate the sciatic nerve. Anyway, as she was talking, I felt total peace from the Holy Spirit and a green light to work with her. She started treating me (the treatment she used was called kinesthetic pain management, which is a practice that increases your awareness of your body, posture, and habits so that you can adjust anything off-kilter), and she worked on me about once a week for over a year. Before she started the treatments, I couldn't sit at all without the pain and nerve irritation making me crazy. On a scale of 1 to 10, it was a 10. But after having the treatments for a period of time my pain went down a lot, and sometimes it's not even noticeable. She is still treating me and I'm still seeing improvement.

The moral of this story: Don't give up in your health journey. You are not too far gone; it's not just because you're "getting older"; there isn't too much junk to clear out. You just have to **start by taking the next step**.

Just as in organizing our houses room by room, I believe that same level of attention should be given to our bodies. First Corinthians 6:19–20 tells us, "Do you not know that **your bodies are temples of the Holy Spirit**, who is in you, whom you have received from God? **You are not your own**; you were bought at a price. Therefore **honor God with your bodies**" (emphasis added). Our bodies are houses for the Holy Spirit. Getting our houses in order applies to our bodies too—nothing hidden, nothing buried. When we take care of our bodies, we are being good stewards of what God has given us and we are better able to be the hands and feet of Christ on the earth.

Maybe we've filled ourselves with junk food over the years, made poor choices, or just haven't made it a priority to take care of ourselves. Maybe we have not allowed our bodies to rest as much as needed. Maybe the image of ourselves is unhealthy, and we need to change the way we think about ourselves. I know it's hard to make changes—it takes intentional planning, new habits, and some sacrifice—but it's worth it. Our bodies need to be taken care of; they need to be restored when they're weak and brought back to health. We need to be good stewards of what we've been given. And remember, health is a journey.

Pause and consider:

Ask the Holy Spirit to lead you into better health. Take a minute with God and go through this inventory, asking Him where you need to get healthy physically.

No Energy / Low Energy / Average Energy / Great Energy

Often Sick / Sometimes Sick / Rarely Sick

Always in Pain / Dull Pain / High Pain

Poor Diet / Average Diet / Healthy Diet

No Exercise / Weekly Exercise / Daily Exercise

1 | When was the last time you felt strong and healthy? What were you doing at the time to make yourself feel that way?

2 | Have you noticed any habits in your life (even if you don't want to give them up) that don't seem to agree with you? What are those?

3 | Take a minute to ask the Holy Spirit if there's anything blocking your overall health and well-being . . . anything that needs to change or be added to your life. Make a note of the things you hear or see.

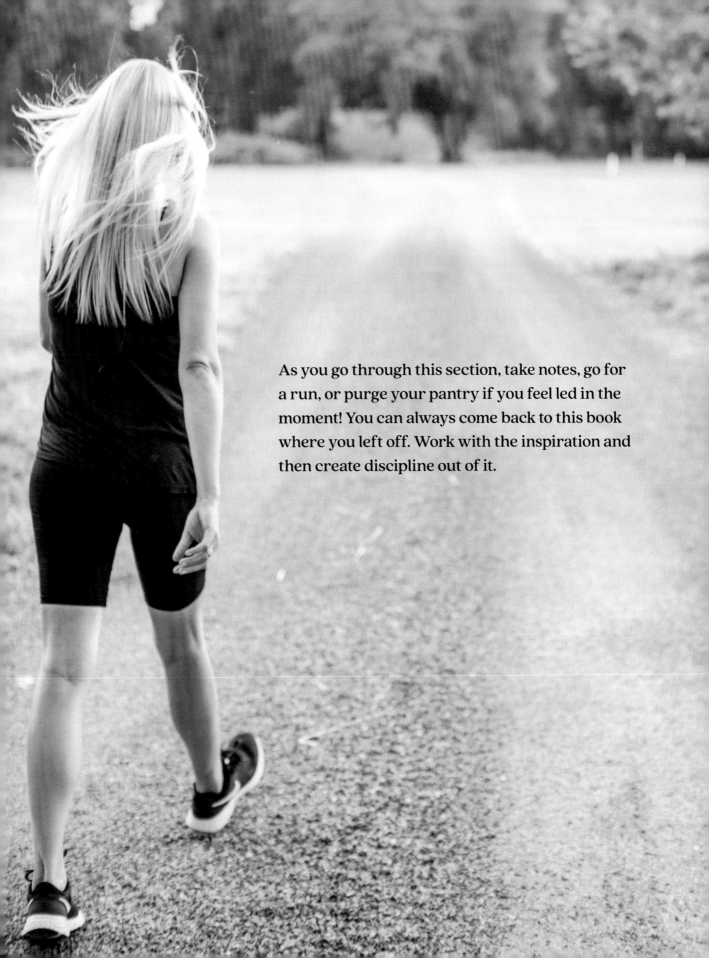

As you go through this section, take notes, go for a run, or purge your pantry if you feel led in the moment! You can always come back to this book where you left off. Work with the inspiration and then create discipline out of it.

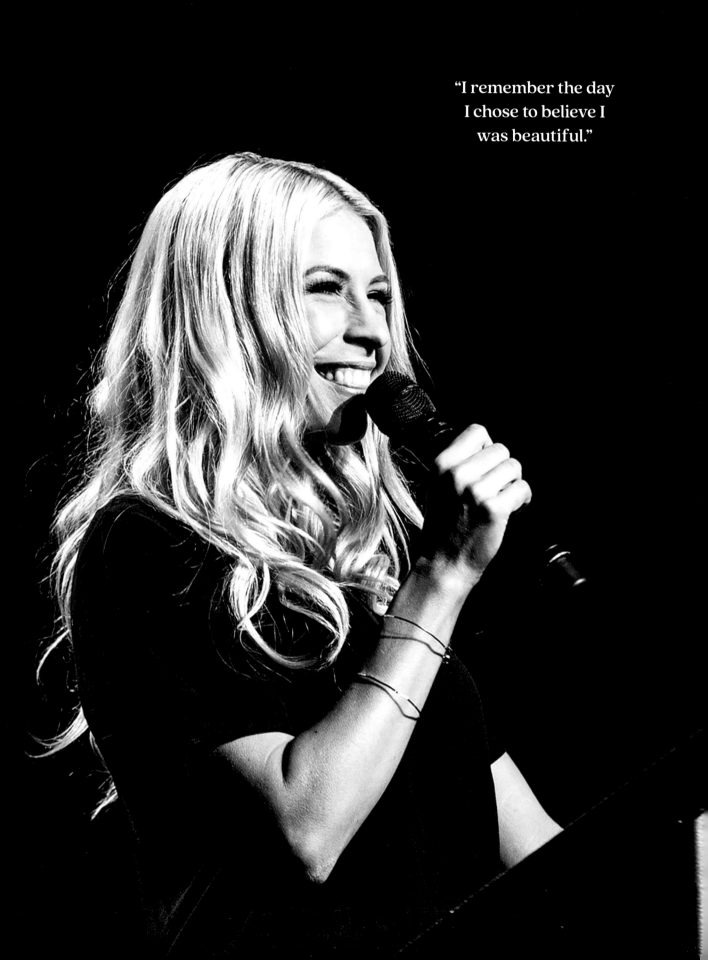

"I remember the day
I chose to believe I
was beautiful."

THE POWER OF BELIEF

Somewhere in the back of our minds, we've collected beliefs about our bodies and where we fall on the "attraction scale." Maybe those beliefs came from things that were said to us—or *not* said.

Maybe our beliefs have taken hold because we think we don't look as good as a friend, not as perfect as that famous Instagrammer, or not as thin as the person in the gym. We build belief systems around ourselves and they bleed into our reality.

I remember the day I chose to believe I was beautiful.

I didn't think I was ugly when I was younger, I just didn't believe I was beautiful. I had a best friend who was better-looking than me, and it wasn't a big deal to me . . . but a reality I accepted. And even though I grew up in a very loving home with incredible parents, verbal affirmation wasn't common around our house. I don't remember being affirmed in my physical beauty much. I know this wasn't an intentional withholding—my parents did a great job raising us, and I felt very loved and cared for.

In my late teens, something began to change in me. I started to think carefully through what I *believed* . . . and got to the root of those beliefs. One of the verses that challenged me was the following:

> There we saw the Nephilim (the sons of Anak, who come from the Nephilim); and we seemed to ourselves like grasshoppers, and so we seemed to them.
>
> *Numbers 13:33* ESV

The context of the verse is that the Israelites had been wandering around the desert for forty years, waiting for their next home. As they approached Canaan—the land God had promised them—Moses sent a group of spies ahead on a scouting mission. These men were supposed to find out what the land was like, how the cities were defended, what strengths and strongholds the locals possessed. Of the twelve spies who went out, ten came back carrying a mixture of truth and exaggeration. The negative exaggeration was that the Israelites were like "grasshoppers" next to the huge men they saw. The intimidation must have made everyone feel insecure and hopeless. And if you look at that verse again in Numbers 13:33, it was surely because *the men believed they were like grasshoppers* next to the giants, and *the giants also looked at them as grasshoppers.*

"You are altogether lovely and you are made in His image."

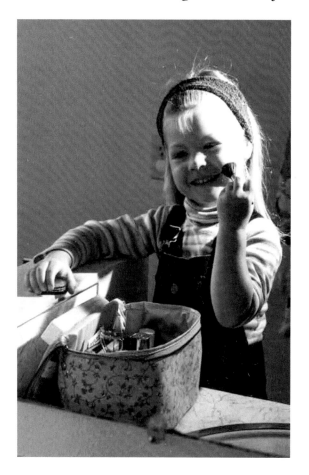

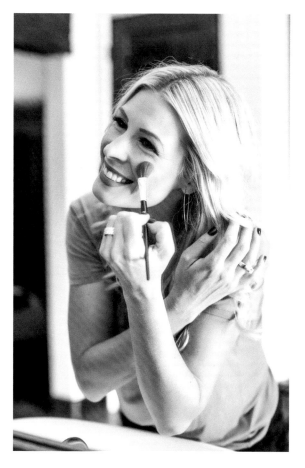

"We seemed to ourselves" became "and so we seemed to them."

So what happened here?

1 │ Their insecurity affected their belief.

2 │ Their belief affected how others saw them.

COMPARISON LEADS TO INSECURITY

When I was a teenager, I often compared myself to other girls around me. Whether it was that they were prettier, thinner, or had better style, I struggled with insecurity and felt like I was lacking in many ways. The grasshopper mentality snuck in; what I believed about myself affected how others viewed me. I didn't believe I was beautiful, so I carried myself as someone who didn't believe she was beautiful. My countenance, confidence, and physical appearance were negatively affected.

Then one day when I was sixteen, I read a verse that I had read many times before, but it hit me in a new way. Don't you love it when God does that?

God created mankind in his own image, in the image of God he created them; male and female he created them.

Genesis 1:27

"God made no mistake when He created you."

What I believe affects my heart, mind, and body, so I don't believe what the world says about me; rather, I want to believe the truth . . . what God says. And the truth is that I am made in God's image! Just like a child is made in the image of his or her parents, we are made in God's image . . . we look like Him. And the more time we spend with Him, we become more like Him, reflecting His love, goodness, beauty, holiness, and grace. The day that verse came to life for me in a new way, I made the intentional choice to agree with what God says about my image and identity: **I am beautiful.**

He has made everything beautiful.

Ecclesiastes 3:11

I am fearfully and wonderfully made.

Psalm 139:14

I can actually look at photos of before and after **my belief changed**, and I can see when I made the intentional choice to agree with what God says. **I can't prove it on paper, but I got better-looking.** My countenance, confidence, and appearance changed because my belief was healthy and in order. I began carrying myself like I believed it. Still, today, when the mirror or the scale shows me something I don't like, I choose to instead believe what God says. I focus on making **healthy choices** and **believing what He says about who I am**.

I believed, so I became. That doesn't mean I don't struggle from time to time; I do.

I still struggle occasionally with my image and my beliefs about my body. After giving birth to three babies, my body changed, and I didn't fit into my teenage-size clothes anymore. I used to think it was that "I gained a few pounds with my pregnancies," but after I had a tummy tuck and thought I would be "smaller" but wasn't, my doctor said, "Honey, you're not a kid anymore . . . Your body has changed and widened to birth your babies." I needed to change my beliefs about my body, because my beliefs at the time weren't grounded in reality. With God's Word guiding me, I began shifting my mind-set to focus on getting healthier instead of on just weight and size.

God made no mistake when He created you. He specifically chose your sex, skin tone, eye color, hair, and body type. **He was not confused when He made you.** He was intentional and knew exactly what He was doing when He knit you together in your mother's womb (see Ps. 139:13). You are altogether lovely and you are made in His image. What would happen if you believed *only* what God was saying about you? You would be transformed, inside and out. Our beliefs impact our bodies and our health. Taking care of your body and getting healthy starts with healthy beliefs about your identity, the body God gave you, and your appearance.

Take time to pause and ask God:

1 | What lies am I believing about myself?

2 | How are my negative, false beliefs impacting my body and my health?

3 | What is God saying about me?

4 | What are you grateful for? Thank God for the body He gave you and all you are able to accomplish. Thank Him for the opportunity to be the hands and feet of Christ on this earth.

The Power of Belief

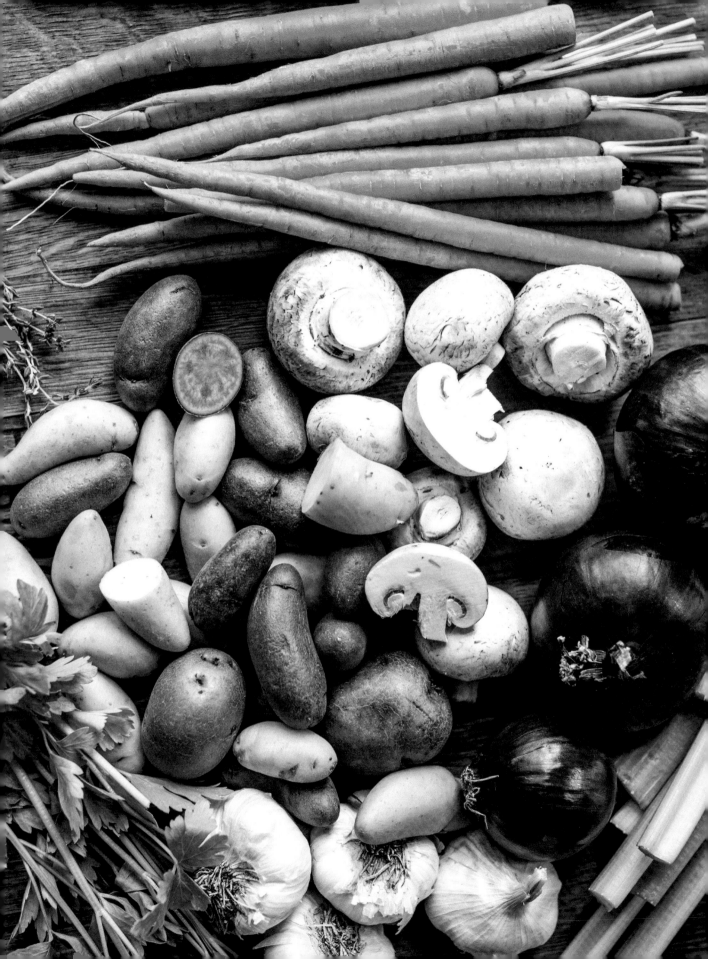

EAT WELL

I've heard it said that "some people eat to live and some live to eat." I'm definitely in that *live-to-eat* category! I usually wake up thinking about delicious food and go to bed dreaming about what we'll eat the next day. I could fill an entire book on this topic (and hopefully will one day). But I'll keep this simple and give you the best tips I've learned along the way—and how we've made eating healthy a priority for our family. With five kids, two working parents, travel, church, lots of hosting, and everything in between, it isn't easy. But as we've learned, if you keep health a priority, no matter what your life looks like, you can *be* healthy.

My mom has always been a great role model for me when it comes to eating well. She has a healthy perspective on her weight and physical appearance. She never obsessed over a certain body size; she taught us to be mindful, exercise, and eat healthy. I don't remember her dieting—she lived with moderation. Like how she would take one bite a day of a Butterfinger, her favorite candy bar, then put it back in the cabinet for another bite or two the next day. (I've followed my mom's lead, but my daily treat most days is a vanilla latte! Heaven!) If my mom ate a ton of carbs one day, the next day she would eat a lot of vegetables and lean meat. She is mindful of what her body needs while not depriving herself of her favorites. It's not about weight or size; rather, it's about health and taking care of the body God has given you.

Wherever you are on your food journey right now, don't feel bad if you're not on a great path yet! I used to drink a lot of Mountain Dew every day and eat McDonald's as well. (Because I worked there, and why is that sausage McMuffin so good?! Get behind me, Satan!) I was not exactly the picture of health. But I've also been on the better side of this where food has become life-giving, healing, and delicious. Now I want to help you on your journey with a few things that helped me.

My top ten tips for getting your food life in order:

1 | **PURGE ALL THE JUNK FOOD.** If you don't have it, you can't eat it. It's as simple as that! Junk food makes you feel gross, does nothing for your energy, causes acne and weight gain, and ultimately depresses you. Plus, corn syrup and foods with chemicals can cause cancer! It's simply not worth putting any of that stuff in your body. Clear out the sugary soda, breakfast cereals, coffee creamer, snacks, and any other food you have that contains chemicals, food colorings, corn syrup, et cetera. Feel free to set this book down right now and purge if you want! I get it, you paid for that stuff, so give it away instead of toss it, but get it out of your house! If you keep it, you or your family will eat it. Big step.

> "Be mindful, exercise, and eat healthy."

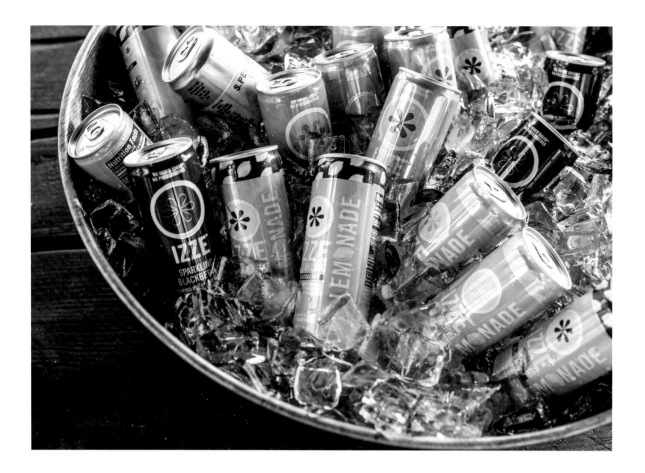

2| **READ FOOD LABELS.** Even if it's not obvious "junk food," you might be surprised at how many items are loaded with sugar and chemicals. For example, standard peanut butter and jelly are *loaded* with sugar. Buy peanut butter that's only peanuts and salt (not the kind that adds sugar), and instead of jelly with added sugar, buy fruit spread that's only fruit.

3| **BUY ORGANIC.** For ultimate health, buy everything organic. Organic produce is better for you because it has a higher production of phytochemicals (minerals and vitamins) and no pesticides. Organic, grass-fed dairy and meat are better for you because the animals are fed nutritiously, and they graze—getting the sun they need. (Eating healthy, exercising, and getting enough sun is vital to animals and humans!) Organic milk has a higher level of omega-3 (which protects against heart disease). Organic meat has less antibiotics and hormones (which are injected into nonorganic meat). And all other organic food (like pasta) is better for you because it has less preservatives. The point is, organic food is safer and has a higher nutritional value.

pro TIP Instead of buying soda, I buy sparkling juice. And instead of chemical coffee creamer, I use half-and-half and agave nectar or organic vanilla syrup.

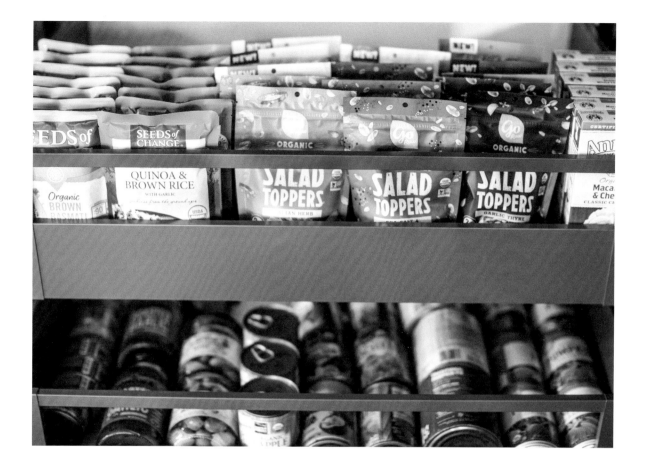

Note: While our family avoids dyes, chemicals, and preservatives, and we eat organic as much as possible—we do eat dairy. I know it's not "good for you," but seriously, God bless butter. When cooking, I try to always use a healthier oil (like coconut oil or olive oil), but when it comes to some things, like popcorn or pancakes, butter is a must. And I'm learning to love vegan butter, thanks to my daughter Haley! What makes me so happy is that now that my kids are older, *they* help *me* to eat healthier.

4 | **SWITCH TO HEALTHIER VERSIONS.**
Love ketchup or soy sauce? Trash the stuff with corn syrup and chemicals and switch to organic. There's plenty out there. The producers of the unhealthy foods are filling them with trash (chemicals, artificial food coloring and sweeteners, fats, sodium nitrite, sugars, high fructose corn syrup, carrageenan, preservatives, trans fats, artificial flavorings, guar gum, MSG, and the like).

5 | **STOCK HEALTHY SNACKS.** I keep tons of options in our fridge and pantry so it's easy for us and our kids to grab quick, healthy snacks. Organic snacks with no sugar (sweetened with fruit juice or coconut sugar), snacks high in protein, and as many pure vegetable and fruit snacks as possible.

6 | **PLAN AHEAD.** If you plan what you'll eat for the day (or the week, if possible), you'll be much more likely to make good choices in the moment. This is especially true if you have kids or busy schedules, because a last-minute meal is an easy target for fast food or heavily processed dinners. You're going to have to think of what's for dinner every night, so why not just plan and get the thinking over in one day? We try to prep and stock on Sundays—with sliced veggies, cooked meat, or tofu—and keep those things in clear glass containers in the fridge so they're ready for breakfast omelets, lunch wraps, and dinner prep during the week.

7 | **USE SUBSCRIPTIONS.** We have monthly subscriptions with Amazon for many household items as well as healthy snacks and drinks. It's an amazing way for our family to save time and money too. And the best part is, you never run out of toilet paper! If you don't need it, just skip the delivery for that month.

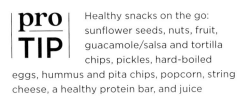

pro TIP Healthy snacks on the go: sunflower seeds, nuts, fruit, guacamole/salsa and tortilla chips, pickles, hard-boiled eggs, hummus and pita chips, popcorn, string cheese, a healthy protein bar, and juice

8 | **EAT WELL ON THE GO TOO.** We're running around and on the road a lot, but yes, even at gas stations you can eat healthy: sunflower seeds, nuts, fruit, guacamole/salsa and tortilla chips, pickles, hard-boiled eggs, hummus and pita chips, popcorn, string cheese, a healthy protein bar, juice, and so on. It's not impossible to eat healthy on the go, you just have to commit to it. **Make the decision that junk food is not an option.** There will always be cheat moments like the corn dog at Disneyland (it's a tradition, even though it wrecks my stomach!) and nachos at a baseball game, but make sure those are moments, not weekly habits. It also helps to have a "not an option" list (for us, that's fast food like McDonald's) so that when you're hungry and craving junk at 10:00 p.m., you've already made the decision to prioritize your health.

9 | **HAVE SELF-CONTROL.** Eating healthy definitely takes self-control (you'll need the Holy Spirit since that's a fruit of His), so ask God for help. "For **God gave us a spirit not of fear but of power and love and self-control**" (2 Tim. 1:7 ESV, emphasis added). With the Holy Spirit, we are able to have self-control, live in a way that's honorable to God, and take care of what He's given us.

10 | **TAKE THE FIRST STEP.** Eating healthy is not all-or-nothing. If your family can't afford to buy all organic food right now, start with one thing, produce or eggs. One step toward health is a victory.

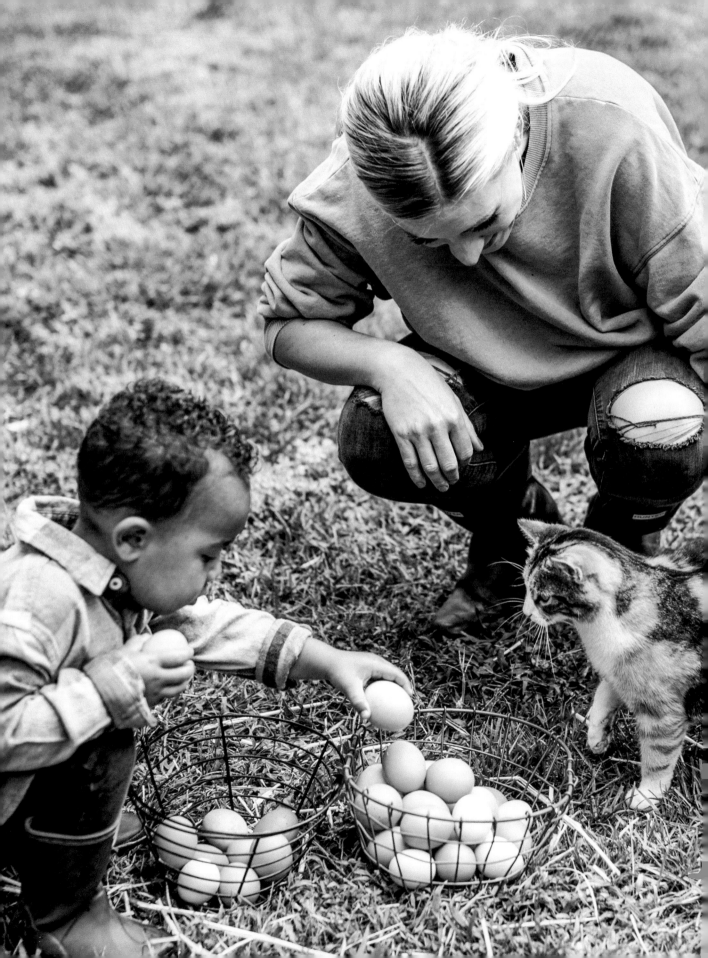

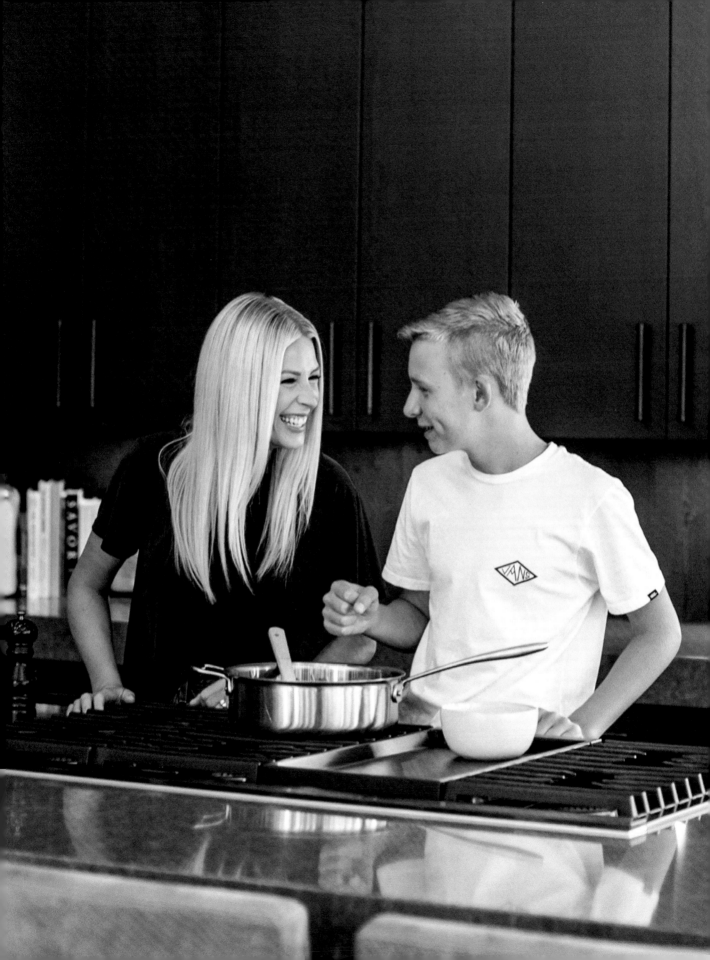

FEEDING KIDS HEALTHY FOOD

From the minute our kids start eating solid food, it's my daily goal to get them to eat healthy (especially more vegetables, using tricks like sneaking blended, steamed cauliflower into their mac 'n' cheese or spinach into smoothies and brownies!). When our oldest daughter was a toddler, I put little bowls on the table with different salad dressings in each one, then told her to dip a bit of lettuce into one dressing at a time to see which one she liked most. She tried them all and ate a whole bowl of lettuce in the process! Her mind was on picking a favorite dressing, not on eating the lettuce. Every time I get my kids to eat vegetables, I feel like I get an imaginary gold star! I'm always looking for creative ways to sneak in more. For example, when I make pasta Bolognese, I chop the veggies really small. Kids are prone to pick out the veggies, but I've found if they're small enough, they'll eat them!

Getting kids to eat vegetables early on, and to try lots of food flavors, develops their palates to enjoy a greater range of tastes as they get older. If your kid seems to be "picky," you have to be the one to help. Kids will eventually eat the healthy stuff, especially if you don't cave and resort to unhealthy replacements when they complain. They'll slowly but surely expand their food choices, and getting them to eat healthy becomes easier.

When our son Ryder was two, I used to cook broccoli for him, and he didn't like it. Then one night we went to a teppanyaki restaurant where they were throwing us raw broccoli to catch in our mouths. Ryder loved that game and he ate a lot of raw broccoli that night! Now at home, when we fake-throw Ryder some raw broccoli, he'll eat a ton! (Whatever works, right?) So try both raw and cooked—you never know what they'll like. Recently, I've been asking, "How loud can you crunch it?" when Ryder is eating carrots and celery. He gets so focused on the noise that he forgets he's eating vegetables!

Not only do I have a priority of teaching my kids *how* to eat healthy, I also train them in how to cook healthy, starting when they're really little. (Plus, following a recipe is *great* math/fraction training!) Just like teaching a child piano lessons, if you teach them a song they love and want to learn, it hooks them with a passion to learn more. I definitely "hook" my kids with making treats (organic and usually pretty healthy with a veggie thrown in). Be careful to not inflict your dislikes onto your kids. Maybe you don't like mushrooms, but that doesn't mean your kids won't. Encourage them to try everything.

It's not always easy in the moment, but make a choice: refuse to let your kids be picky and expand their palates. Even if it is organic, an everyday diet of mac 'n' cheese, chicken nuggets, and fruit snacks isn't going to cut it. (I do have a great recipe for healthy chicken nuggets on page 106.)

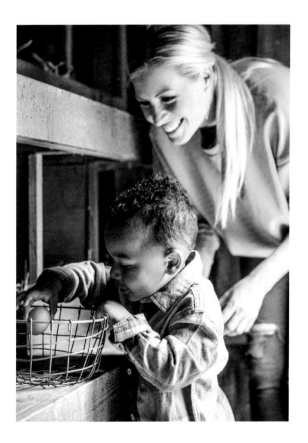

Baked Chicken Nuggets
and Dipping Sauce

PANKO MIX

2 cups panko bread crumbs (or gluten-free panko)

Olive oil cooking spray

2 teaspoons poultry seasoning

1 teaspoon black pepper

2 teaspoons salt

1 teaspoon dried rosemary

1 teaspoon garlic powder

1 teaspoon onion powder

EGG MIXTURE

4 eggs

4 tablespoons milk (or almond milk)

1 teaspoon hot sauce (our family fave is Crystal)

MEAT MIXTURE

2 pounds ground chicken or turkey

2 teaspoons salt

1 teaspoon black pepper

Heat the oven to 400°F. Spread the panko bread crumbs evenly on a baking sheet and coat the layer with olive oil cooking spray. Bake for 2 minutes. Stir and bake 2 more minutes. Put the toasted panko in a bowl and add the poultry seasoning, black pepper, salt, rosemary, garlic powder, and onion powder. Mix well.

In a separate bowl, whisk together the eggs, milk, and hot sauce.

In a third bowl, combine the ground chicken or turkey, salt, and pepper.

Coat the baking sheet with olive oil spray and set an oven-safe wire rack on top of it. With a small scoop, make a ball of the meat mixture and place it into the egg mixture. Coat well and then dredge the ball in the panko mixture and flatten it slightly to make a nugget shape. Place the nuggets an inch apart on the wire rack. Spray the nuggets with olive oil. Bake about 20 minutes, or until the chicken reaches 165°F. Serve with dipping sauces and celery on the side.

Buffalo Dipping Sauce

1 cup hot sauce

½ cup butter, melted

¼ teaspoon garlic powder

½ teaspoon salt

Put all ingredients together, mix, and dip!

Creamy Honey Mustard BBQ

Mix together equal parts of your favorite barbecue sauces, avocado (or regular) mayo, and honey mustard.

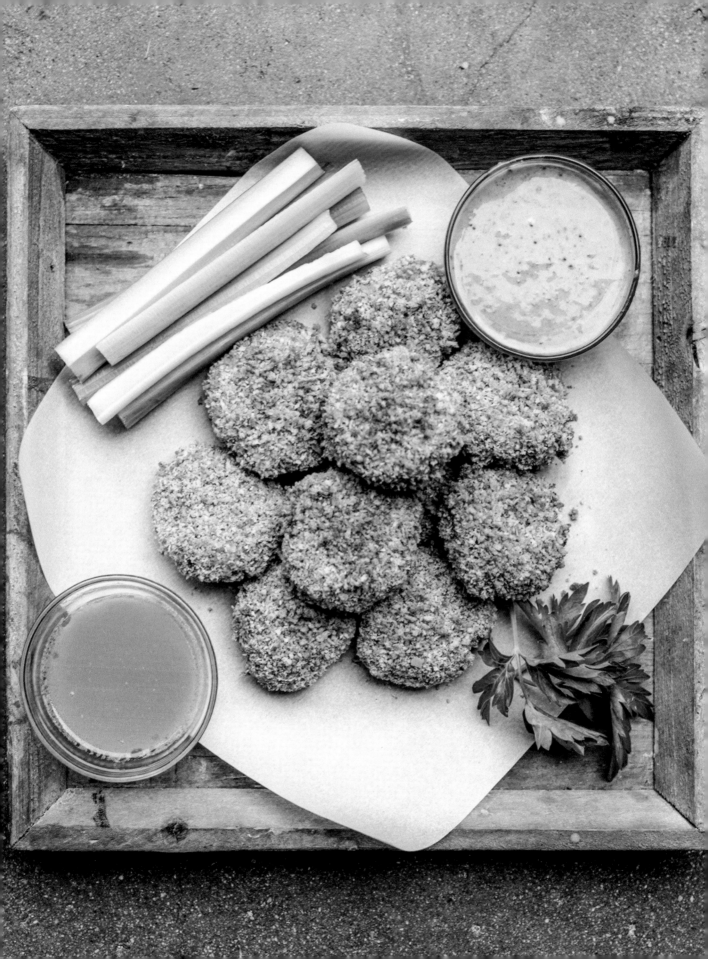

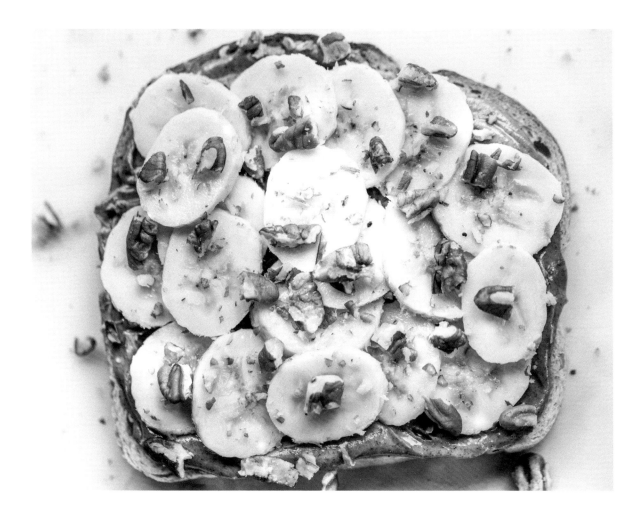

Here are some ideas to swap out unhealthy options for healthy ones: For breakfast, instead of a plain bagel and cream cheese, try a sprouted whole wheat bagel with veggie cream cheese or avocado toast! Try steel-cut oats with lots of topping options (berries, bananas, dried fruit, honey, coconut, cocoa nibs, nuts, chia seeds) instead of sugar-filled instant oatmeal packs. Cereal made with honey is a great option, especially granola. (Use honey instead of sugar as a sweetener when you can. Honey is the only sweetener that has nutritional value.) Other great options: plain yogurt and honey instead of sugary yogurts (yogurt has great probiotics), or a smoothie with almond milk, frozen fruit, plain yogurt, and honey. And whether it's oatmeal and nuts or puréed pumpkin added to a cookie, I always try to add nutritious ingredients even into sweets.

Really, there are so many healthy options and alternatives out there, it's just a matter of purging the junk and getting into a new routine! (For more great ideas, try reading Jessica Seinfeld's book, *Deceptively Delicious*.)

The point is, if you get your kids eating healthy and trying new things, they'll develop a taste for healthy food and build their own healthy habits. And teach them the "why" behind eating healthy and their need for the Holy Spirit to help them with self-control!

SNACKS AND PACKED LUNCHES

We keep snack drawers filled with healthy options that the kids can get by themselves for snacking and lunch packing. School mornings in our house can look a lot like that scene from *Home Alone* where they wake up late and mad-dash to the airport, so our kids pack their lunches the night before.

Our simple lunch packing rule: Pack at least five items. Include one vegetable (even if that's pickles, olives, hummus, or dried seaweed); at least one item with protein; and water. (Dehydration is too common, especially in kids.) And yes, we sneak in a few nonhealthy items sometimes.

Some of our favorite snacks/lunch packing ideas:

- Roasted, salted nuts and seeds: peanuts, cashews, almonds, pecans, sunflower seeds

- Toasted sesame-flavored dried seaweed

- Fruit and vegetable puree packs (get those veggies in whenever and wherever you can!)

- Fruit and vegetable fruit snacks

- A banana and a nut butter packet (sweetened with honey)

- Veggie straws

- Fruit and nut bars

- Potato chips

- Crackers with chicken salad

- Popcorn

- Cheesy corn puffs

- Tortilla chips with salsa or guacamole

- Hummus and carrots (or hummus and grilled chicken)

- Olives

- Organic meat sticks

- Curried chicken salad

- Gyro (pita, meat, hummus, tzatziki, lettuce, tomatoes)

- Bistro box (grapes, cheese, crackers, baby carrots, almonds, pickles)

- Chicken Caesar salad (toppings and dressing on the side so it doesn't get soggy)

- Pickles

- Asian rice bowls (rice, avocado, meat or tofu, cilantro, spicy mayo, sesame seeds, green onion, sesame seed oil, rice wine vinegar)

- Mexican rice bowl (rice, meat or tofu, beans, salsa, avocado, cilantro, lime, jalapeños, green onions)

- Turkey sandwich (with arugula, pesto, or mustard)

- Spinach wraps with turkey, avocado, tomato, bell peppers, banana peppers, spinach, garlic powder, salt, and pepper

- Bean-and-cheese burrito

- Chili

- Spicy sesame edamame (page 116)

- Hard-boiled eggs or deviled eggs (page 129)

- Buffalo chicken (canned organic chicken with buffalo sauce mixed in) sandwich with celery sticks on the side

- Healthy PBJ (organic fruit spread and no-sugar peanut butter)

- Celery, peanut butter, and raisins ("ants on a log")

- Pasta salad (made with veggie pasta)

- Berries with yogurt and honey

- Apple nachos (chopped green apple with peanut butter, raisins, honey, cocoa nibs, and dried coconut)

- Watermelon with fresh lime juice

- Organic juice boxes (no sugar added)

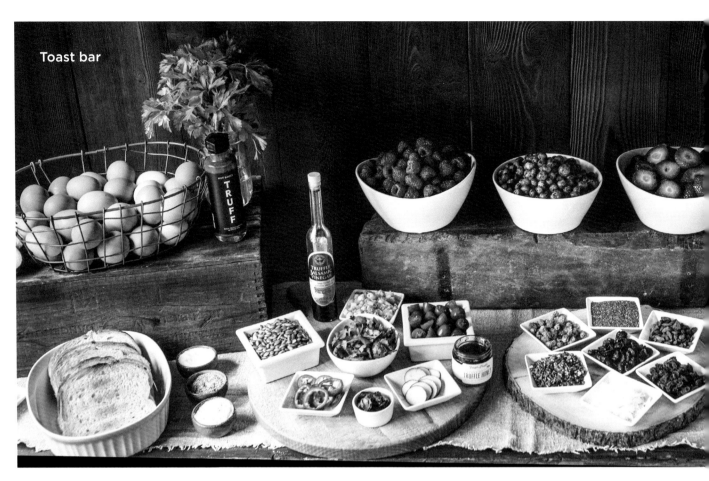

Toast bar

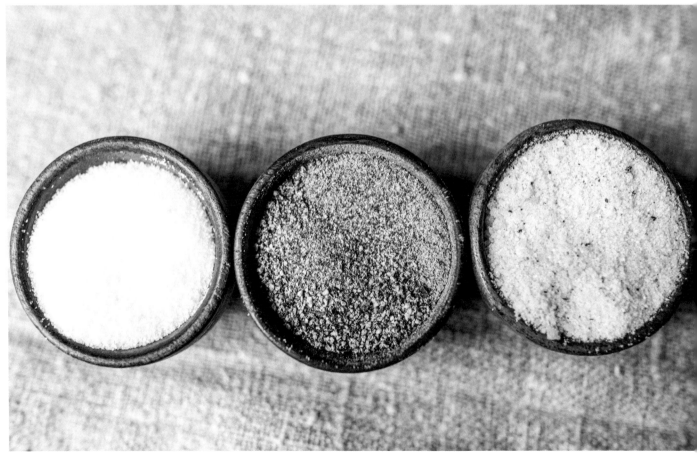

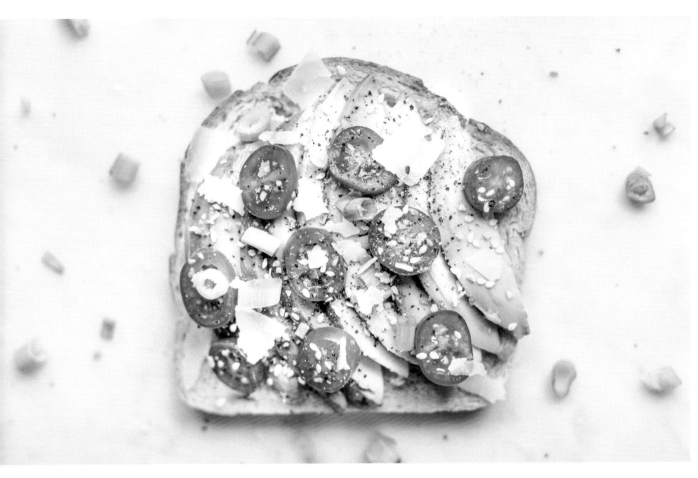

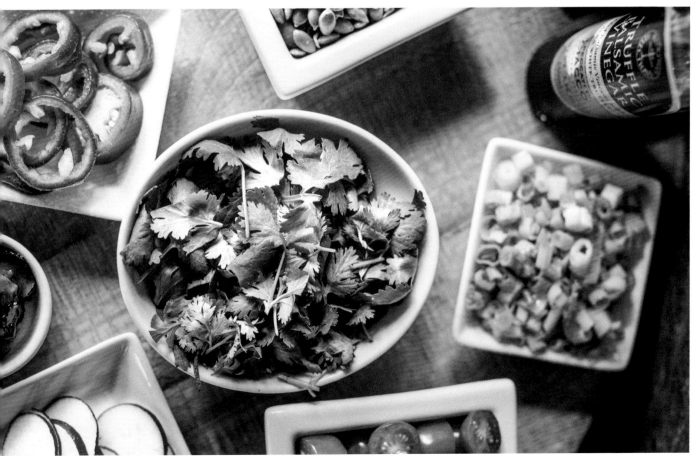

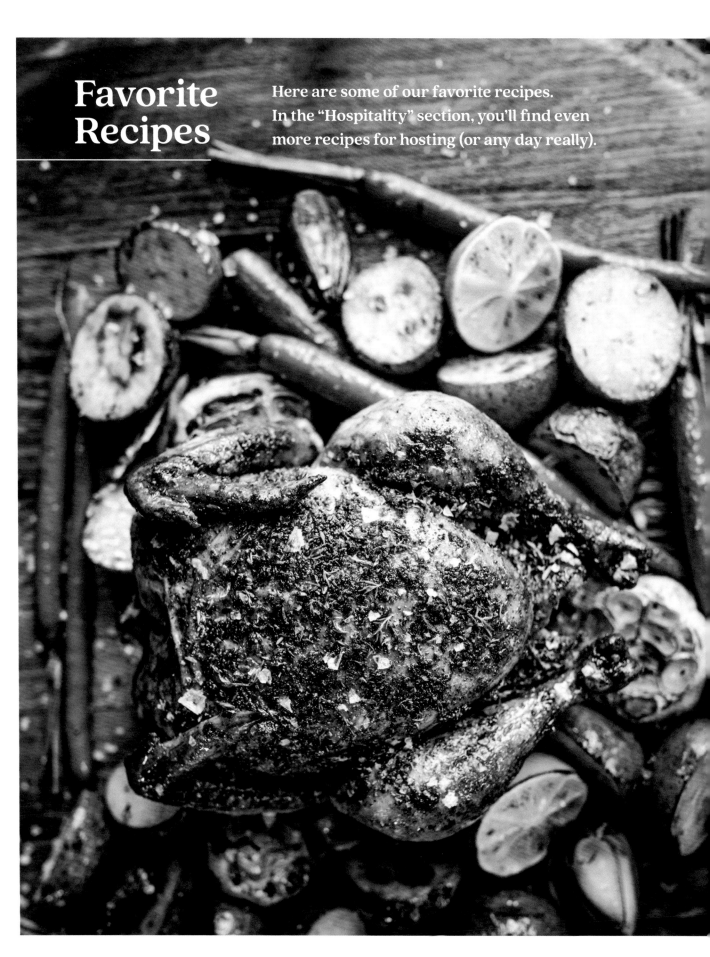

Favorite Recipes

Here are some of our favorite recipes. In the "Hospitality" section, you'll find even more recipes for hosting (or any day really).

Roast Chicken

2 pounds baby carrots

6 whole garlic bulbs, cut in half horizontally

1 large onion, peeled and sliced in half

20 small potatoes (I don't peel these because potato skins are good for you!)

4 stalks celery, cut into 1-inch pieces

½ cup extra-virgin olive oil

1 tablespoon salt

2 teaspoons lemon pepper

1 teaspoon rosemary

1 teaspoon thyme

1 (5-pound) chicken

2 tablespoons soy sauce

2 tablespoons butter, melted

1-2 tablespoons lemon juice

3 tablespoons fresh parsley, chopped

Preheat the oven to 425°F. Place the carrots, garlic, onion, potatoes, and celery on a large baking sheet.

Whisk together the olive oil, salt, lemon pepper, rosemary, and thyme. Pour over the vegetables and mix with your hands. Place the chicken on top of the layer of vegetables.

Mix the soy sauce with the melted butter and brush over the chicken. Put the baking sheet in the oven and roast about 60 minutes, or until the internal temperature of the chicken reaches 165°F.

Finish with a squeeze of lemon juice over the chicken and sprinkle with fresh chopped parsley and salt and pepper to taste.

To take your chicken to the next level, brine it first (two-day process).

Brine

4 lemons, cut in half

6 bay leaves

1 bunch of fresh parsley

1 bunch of fresh thyme

¼ cup honey

1 bulb garlic, cut in half horizontally

⅛ cup black peppercorns

1 cup salt

1 gallon water

Combine all the ingredients and bring the brine to a boil. Once boiling, remove from heat. Pour the brine into a large container (I use a huge stockpot). Chill in the refrigerator.

When the brine is cool, add the chicken and chill in the refrigerator for 12 hours. Take the chicken out and dry with paper towels. Strain the brine down the sink and toss what's left in the strainer. Place the chicken back in the pot and leave uncovered in the refrigerator for 24 to 48 hours, to dry. Then remove the chicken from the refrigerator and set aside for 1 to 2 hours so it comes to room temperature.

Beef Stew

2 pounds beef stew meat (cut into 1-inch pieces)

Salt and freshly ground black pepper

3 tablespoons extra-virgin olive oil

2 medium onions, peeled and cut into 1-inch pieces

7 garlic cloves, peeled and minced

1½ tablespoons tomato paste

¼ cup all-purpose flour

2 cups dry red wine

46 ounces beef broth

2 cups water

1 bay leaf

½ teaspoon fresh thyme

20 baby carrots, cut into 1-inch pieces on a diagonal

1½ pounds small potatoes, cut in half

4 celery stalks, thinly sliced

8 mushrooms, sliced

Fresh parsley, chopped (for serving)

Preheat the oven to 325°F.

Dry the beef with a paper towel and season generously on both sides with salt and pepper. In a large Dutch oven, heat 1 tablespoon of the olive oil over medium-high heat. Add the meat and brown for about 5 minutes. (To sear the meat, don't crowd the pan and let the meat get a nice brown crust before turning with tongs.) Scoop the meat out with a slotted spoon, leaving the juices in the pot, and place the meat on a plate. Cut off any large pieces of fat and discard.

Add the onion and garlic to the pot and sauté for about 5 minutes, stirring and scraping the brown bits from the bottom of the pan. Add the tomato paste and cook for a minute more. Add the beef with its juices back to the pan and sprinkle with the flour. Stir until the flour is dissolved, 1 to 2 minutes. Add the wine and stir again to loosen any brown bits from the bottom of the pan.

Next add the beef broth, water, bay leaf, and thyme. Bring to a boil. Then add the carrots, potatoes, celery, and mushrooms. Cover with a lid and transfer to the oven for 2 to 3 hours, until the vegetables are cooked and the meat is tender. Remove the bay leaf and toss it. Taste and add more salt and pepper, if needed. Garnish with fresh parsley.

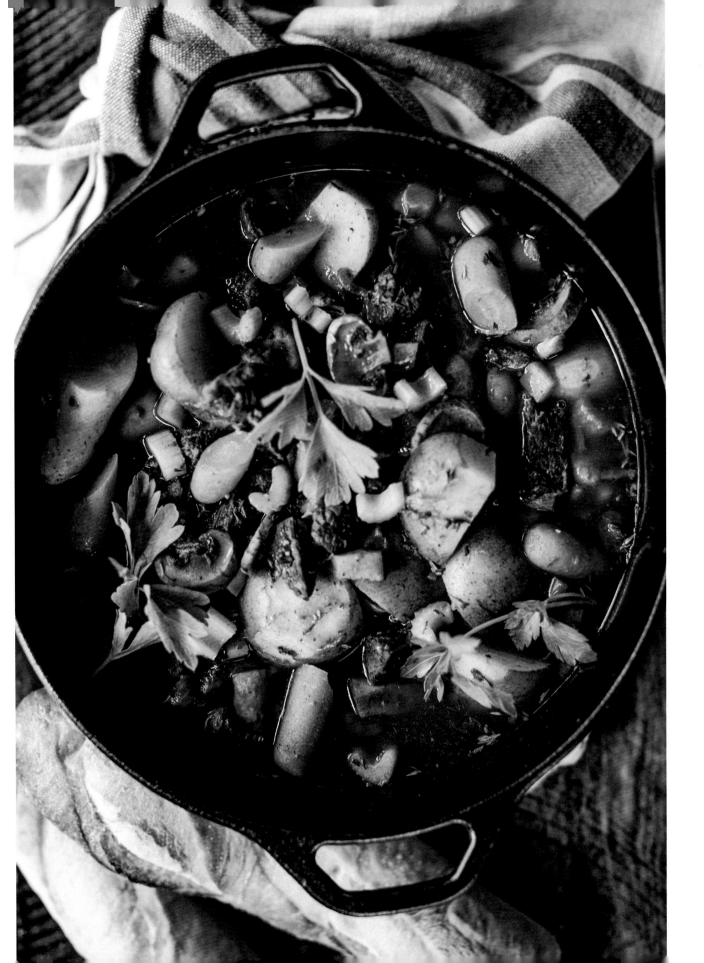

Spicy Edamame

1 pound edamame
beans in the shell

¼ cup toasted
sesame oil

Shichimi togarashi
(a spicy Japanese
red chili blend)

Salt and black
pepper

You can buy cooked edamame or raw. If raw, just follow the instructions on the package to boil them. If frozen, bring a large pot of generously salted water to a boil. Add the edamame, return to a boil, and cook until bright green, 3 to 5 minutes. Drain.

Place the edamame in a large bowl and pour the toasted sesame oil over the top. Toss until coated.

Then sprinkle with shichimi togarashi, salt, and black pepper to taste.

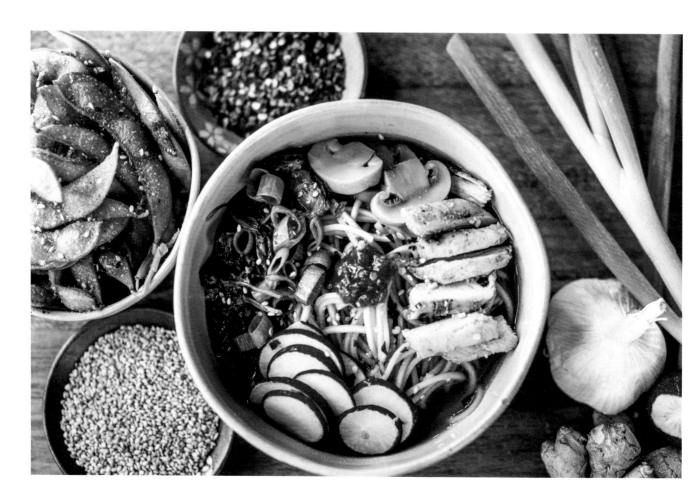

Health

Ramen

CHICKEN MARINADE

2 tablespoons mirin

2 tablespoons soy sauce

¼ teaspoon cayenne pepper

2 garlic cloves, peeled and finely chopped

4 boneless skinless chicken breasts

BROTH

5 cups chicken broth

4 green onions, chopped

5 garlic cloves, peeled and minced

2-inch piece of fresh ginger, peeled and thinly sliced

½ teaspoon red pepper flakes

¼ cup light soy sauce

¼ cup mirin

6 ounces mushrooms, sliced

13 ounces dried ramen noodles

GREENS

2 handfuls of spinach and/or 4 baby bok choy

1 teaspoon soy sauce

1 teaspoon sesame oil

1 teaspoon minced garlic

RAMEN TOPPINGS

4 green onions, finely sliced

Sliced radishes or bean sprouts

Chili garlic oil

Toasted sesame seeds

Place all ingredients for the chicken marinade in a bowl and mix well. Coat the chicken and let it marinate for at least 1 hour in the refrigerator.

Preheat the oven to 425°F and line a baking sheet with parchment paper. Place the chicken on the baking sheet and put it in the oven for 15 minutes. After 15 minutes, flip the chicken over and let it cook for another 10 to 15 minutes. Remove the baking sheet from the oven and let the chicken cool. Slice the chicken and set aside.

Place the broth, onion, garlic, ginger, red pepper flakes, soy sauce, and mirin in a saucepan. Stir and cover the pot. Let it come to a boil at medium to high heat. Then simmer for 25 minutes. Taste and add more soy sauce if needed. Add the mushrooms and let them cook for about 3 minutes. (If you don't like mushrooms, you can add a tablespoon of mushroom powder to the broth.) Next, add the dry noodles to the broth and cook for 3 to 4 minutes.

Rinse the greens and place them in a skillet. Add the soy sauce, sesame oil, and garlic. Cook on medium-high for 3 to 5 minutes.

Then, make your ramen bowl the way you like! Scoop some ramen and broth into your bowl. Top with chicken, greens, green onion, radishes, chili garlic oil, or toasted sesame seeds.

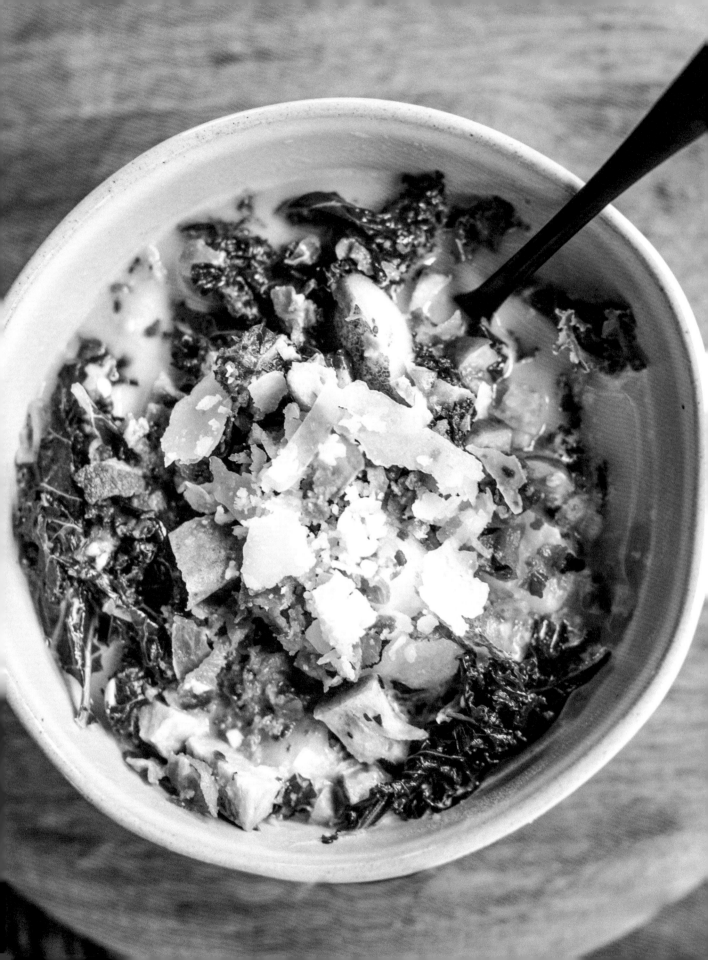

Potato, Sausage, and Kale Soup

6 ounces bacon, chopped

1 tablespoon extra-virgin olive oil

1 pound sausage (I use organic chicken or pork sausage)

1 medium onion, finely diced

10 large garlic cloves, peeled and minced

4 cups chicken broth

6 cups water

5 medium potatoes, peeled and cut in half

2 bunches of kale, stems removed and torn into pieces and rinsed

1 cup heavy whipping cream

Salt and freshly ground black pepper

Fresh Parmesan cheese, to serve

Buttered sourdough baguette, to serve

In a large pot over medium-high heat, sauté the chopped bacon until browned. Transfer the cooked bacon to a plate. Add about 1 tablespoon of oil to the pot to coat the bottom.

Add the sausage and stir, breaking it up, until cooked through. Take out the cooked sausage and add it to the plate.

Add the onion to the pot. Sauté until soft and then add the minced garlic and sauté a minute. Add the broth and water, and bring the mixture to a boil. Add the potatoes and cook until easily pierced with a fork (10 to 12 minutes). When potatoes are almost done, add chopped kale and cooked sausage and bring everything to a boil.

Stir in the cream and bring back to a boil. Season to taste with salt and freshly ground black pepper, then remove from heat. Sprinkle the soup with bacon and grated Parmesan.

Serve with slices of buttered sourdough baguette.

Kale Chips

4 bunches of kale

2 cups raw cashews

2 tablespoons minced garlic

1 large bell pepper, cored and seeds removed

2 tablespoons fresh lemon juice

5 tablespoons nutritional yeast

1 teaspoon salt

¼ teaspoon black pepper

1 tablespoon agave nectar

1 teaspoon cayenne pepper

Wash the kale and remove the stems. Tear the kale into big pieces and place in a large bowl.

Submerge the cashews in filtered water and let them soak for 2 to 4 hours, or until soft.

Drain the cashews. Add the soaked cashews, garlic, bell pepper, lemon juice, yeast, salt, black pepper, agave nectar, and cayenne to a food processor and blend until smooth. With a spatula, pour the blended mixture onto the kale and mix with your hands (I use gloves) until the pieces are evenly coated.

Place the kale pieces on dehydrator racks and dehydrate for 12 hours at 105°F.

NOTE: I use a dehydrator for these—because it gets them crispy and completely dried out. (You can find one for about $40 if you want to make the investment!) If you don't have a dehydrator, you can bake them in the oven at 350°F for 10 to 15 minutes.

pro TIP

As mentioned above, you can put the kale chips in the oven, but it's best to use a dehydrator! It makes them extra crispy.

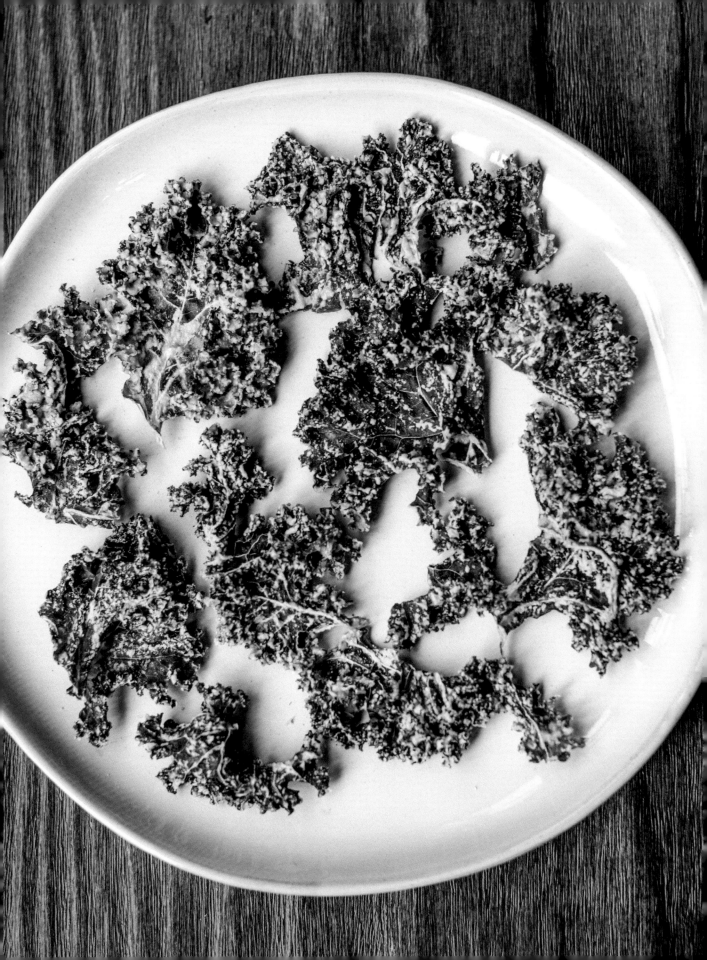

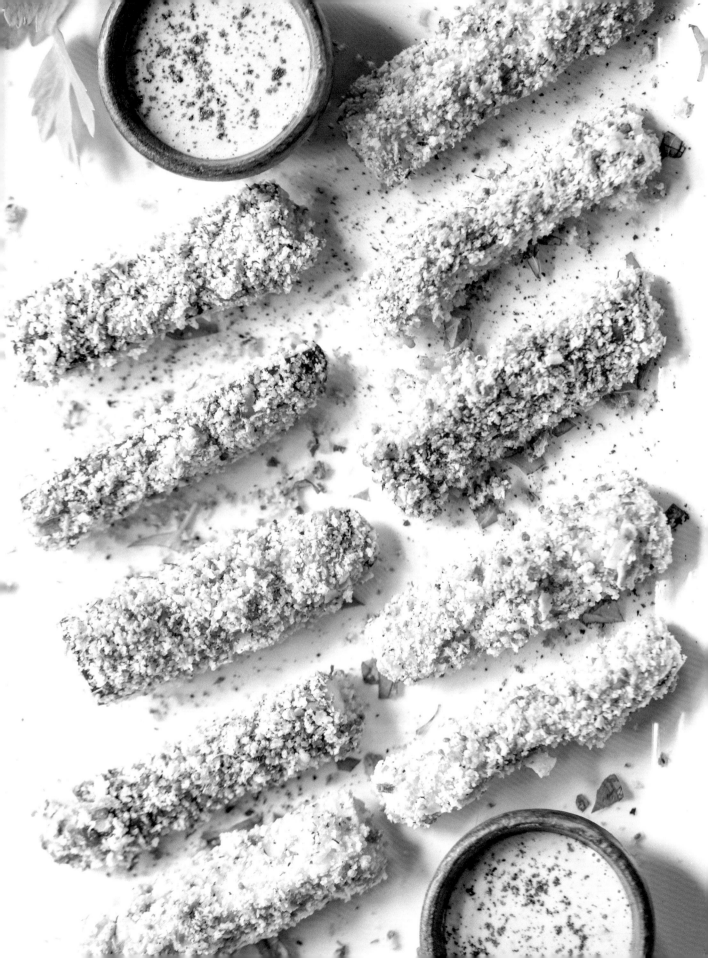

Zucchini Fries

3 cups panko bread crumbs

1½ cups fresh Parmesan cheese, shredded

3 teaspoons Italian seasoning

1½ teaspoons salt

1½ teaspoons freshly ground black pepper

1 cup all-purpose flour

5 large eggs, beaten

8 large zucchini, quartered lengthwise

4 tablespoons chopped fresh parsley

Fresh basil

Cayenne pepper

Preheat the oven to 425°F. Coat a cooling rack with nonstick spray and place on a baking sheet; set aside.

In a large bowl (or plastic bag), combine the panko bread crumbs, Parmesan cheese, Italian seasoning, salt, and pepper. Put the flour in a separate bowl or bag; in a third bowl or bag, add the eggs. Working in batches, dredge the zucchini in flour, dip into the eggs, then dredge in the panko mixture, pressing to coat.

Place the zucchini on the cooling rack that's on the baking sheet. Place in the oven and bake for about 20 minutes, or until crisp.

Serve immediately sprinkled with parsley, basil, and cayenne pepper, to taste.

Dipping Sauce

½ cup fresh dill

½ cup fresh mint

½ cup fresh parsley

⅓ cup fresh basil

2 whole peeled garlic cloves

3 green onions, trimmed

1½ tablespoons fresh lemon juice

Salt and black pepper

½ cup extra-virgin olive oil

½ cup feta cheese

½ cup Greek yogurt

¼ cup mayonnaise

Combine all ingredients in a blender and pulse until combined. God bless appliances doing the hard work for you!

Breakfast Taco

1 package corn tortillas

1 (16-ounce) can refried beans

1 bunch of cilantro, finely chopped

1 bunch of green onions, finely chopped

1 (12-ounce) jar jalapeños (regular or tamed), sliced

1 block cotija (or your favorite) cheese, crumbled

3 avocados, pitted and sliced

6 eggs

Chipotle Aioli (below)

Hot sauce

Salt and pepper

Preheat the oven to 350°F. Wrap the tortillas in a packet of aluminum foil and bake for 15 to 20 minutes, until heated through. (I like to make aluminum packets of 5 to 6 tortillas in each, so that when serving, half will stay hot in the foil.)

Next, empty a can of refried beans into a microwave-safe bowl and cover. Warm in the microwave. Place cilantro, green onions, jalapeños, cotija cheese, and avocados in separate small bowls.

Scramble the eggs and remove them from the heat, but keep them in the pan so they stay warm.

Let people make their tacos the way they like. Serve all the fresh toppings, along with chipotle aioli, hot sauce, salt, and pepper on the side.

Chipotle Aioli

1 cup mayonnaise

2 tablespoons finely chopped chives

2 garlic cloves, peeled and minced

2 teaspoons fresh lime juice

1 teaspoon chipotle chile powder

Salt and pepper

Whisk together the ingredients, then chill until ready to serve.

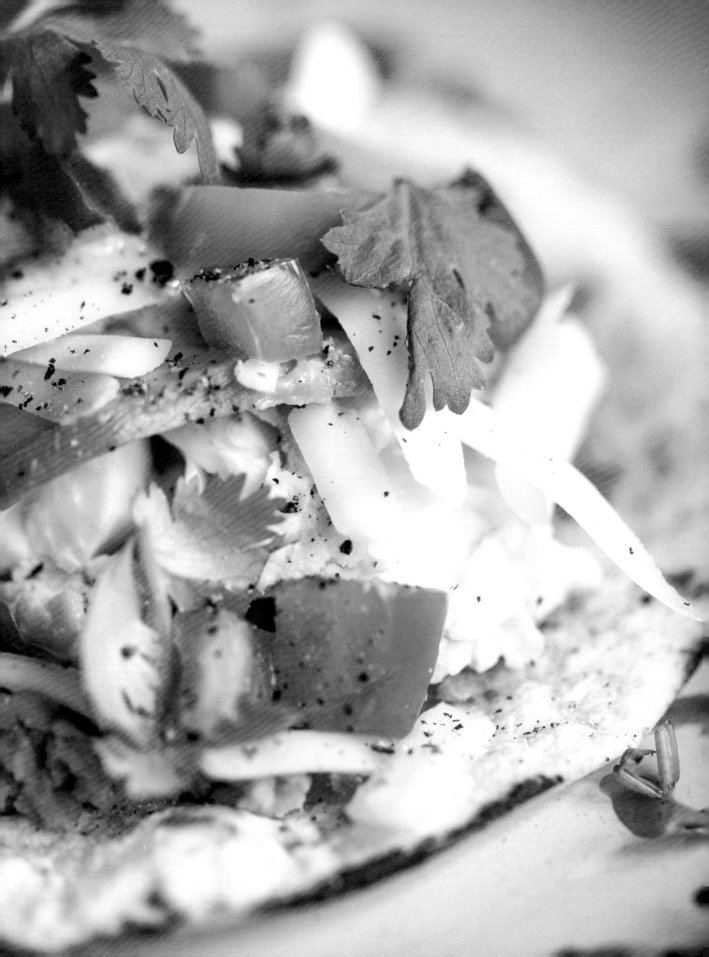

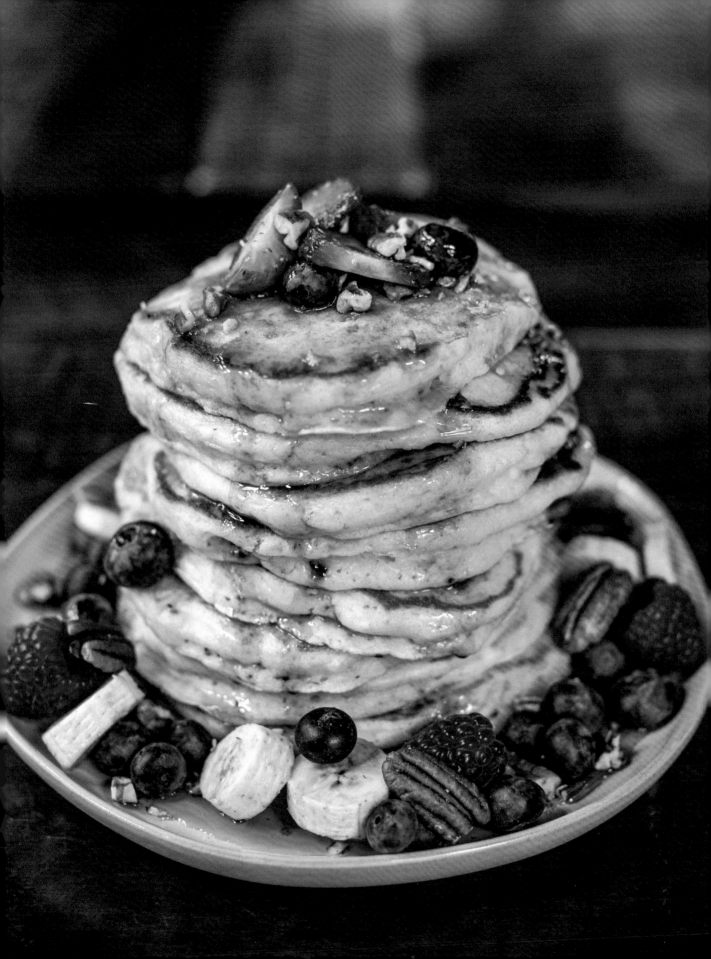

Greek Yogurt Pancakes

1½ cups Greek (or cashew) yogurt

6 tablespoons salted butter, melted

3 eggs

3 cups whole (or oat) milk

1 teaspoon bourbon vanilla extract (or regular vanilla extract)

4½ cups all-purpose (or gluten-free) flour

1½ tablespoons baking powder

¾ teaspoon baking soda

1 teaspoon salt

Optional: blueberries

Butter, maple syrup, peanut butter, chopped pecans, berries, and whipped cream (for serving)

Whisk the yogurt, butter, eggs, milk, and bourbon vanilla extract in a large bowl. In a separate bowl, sift together the flour, baking powder, baking soda, and salt. Then combine the wet and dry ingredients.

Scoop the batter onto a hot, buttered griddle or pan over medium-high heat. Flip when tiny bubbles form on the edges of the pancake. (If you're adding blueberries, sprinkle them on before flipping.) Cook about a minute longer on the other side until golden brown.

Serve with lots of butter and garnishes such as maple syrup, peanut butter, chopped pecans, berries, and whipped cream.

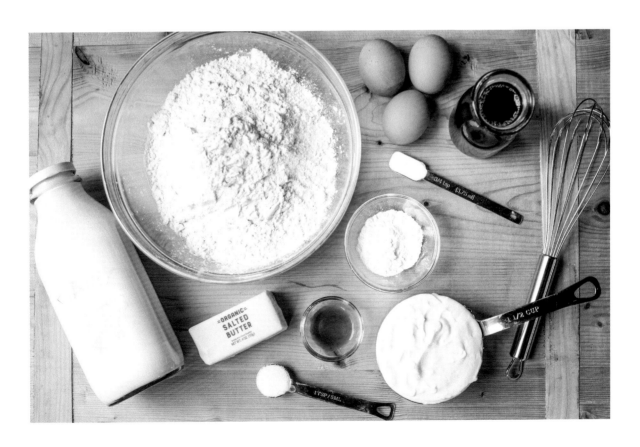

Your Body

Apple and Pecan Salad
with Crumbled Blue Cheese

1 head green leaf lettuce, chopped or torn

½ cup dried cranberries

½ cup chopped pecans

2 whole apples, cored and thinly sliced

¼ cup olive oil

1 tablespoon Dijon mustard

1 tablespoon maple syrup

1 teaspoon apple cider vinegar

Salt and freshly ground black pepper

6 ounces blue cheese, crumbled (I prefer Point Reyes)

Add the lettuce, cranberries, pecans, and apples to a large salad bowl.

In a separate container (I use a mason jar with a lid), add the olive oil, mustard, maple syrup, vinegar, and salt and pepper to taste. Then shake well or whisk together.

Pour a little of the salad dressing over the top of the salad and toss to combine. Top with blue cheese crumbles, or leave the blue cheese on the side for people to add if they want.

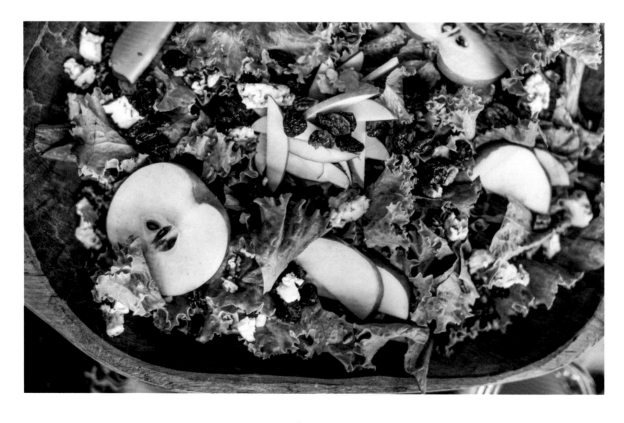

Truffle and Bacon Deviled Eggs

6 eggs, hard-boiled (I buy mine from Costco because they're perfect and peeled)

2 tablespoons mayonnaise or avocado mayonnaise

1 teaspoon Dijon mustard

½ teaspoon fresh lemon juice

White or black truffle oil to taste

2 teaspoons minced green onion, plus additional for garnish

6 strips of cooked bacon, chopped in pieces

Salt and freshly ground black pepper

Slice the hard-boiled eggs in half vertically and scoop the egg yolks into a blender. Add the mayonnaise, mustard, and lemon juice and blend until smooth and fluffy. Add the truffle oil, green onion, and salt and pepper to taste; pulse until blended.

Using a piping bag (or a plastic bag with the corner snipped off), fill each egg white half with the truffle mixture from the blender. Sprinkle with green onion, bacon, salt, and pepper.

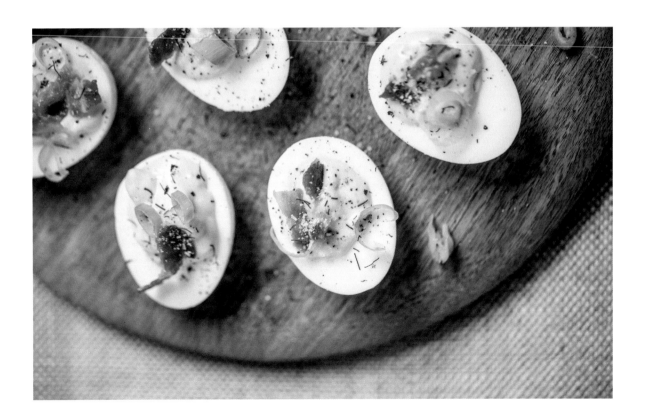

EXERCISE

Exercise is vital not only for your weight management; it's vital for your whole body, especially your mental health. It reduces stress, improves your mood, gives you energy, and releases endorphins! So, when you get home from work and just want to crash? Don't! Go for a walk or do a workout!

I know adding daily exercise to your life can be a big shift to make, but it's one of those things that, once you do it, the energy and how you feel will speak for itself. The key is, you have to find what works for you, because it's a commitment. Is working out/walking in the morning or at night better for you? Whatever works for you, do it. To make sure I stay on track (because, like many of you, I have a lot on my plate and exercise can easily get ditched), I've found three things that help me keep exercise a priority:

1 | **PUT EXERCISE ON YOUR CALENDAR—** just like you would a meeting or an appointment. This might sound like a small step, but when you get the calendar alert, it seriously helps! It could be for a fifteen-minute stretching session or a one-hour bike ride with a pull-behind kid carrier. If you make it a calendar event, you're more likely to do it.

2 | **REPLACE COFFEE DATES OR WORK MEETINGS WITH A WALK.** Instead of sitting around at tables and consuming calories, walk some calories off with your friend, coworker, or the person you're counseling. You can also make a long walk part of your date with your spouse!

3 | **FIND WHAT WORKS FOR YOU.** Hate the gym? Me too. But if the gym works for you, do it! If you decide running trails is better than a treadmill, go for it. Just choose. Having someone meet you for a walk or at the gym is also great accountability. I like long morning walks, sometimes by myself (praying, listening to an audio Bible, or simply enjoying being able to think straight before my wild day begins), or with a friend, kids, or my husband. We love the time together. It lifts our moods and we get a great workout too!

Speaking of kids, get your kids to be active! It's so easy for them to be indoors and on their phones or games all day. They are sitting down in school a lot already, and the more active they are, the healthier they are physically and emotionally. Many times, kids act out because of too much sugar and not enough exercise. The more they can be outdoors, getting fresh air, playing, doing sports, or exercising, the better. Teaching them regular discipline helps them develop healthy patterns for later in their lives. They learn how much better their bodies feel after exercising, and just like healthy food habits, they will start to exercise without being asked.

I know sometimes we have physical limits, and maybe a certain exercise is not in our best interest. This goes back to paying attention to your body and seeking medical advice if something feels off. But don't use your limits as an excuse to give up. Just find an alternative and go for it!

Hebrews 12:1–2 says, "Throw off everything that hinders and the sin that so easily entangles. And let us **run with perseverance** the race marked out for us, fixing our eyes on Jesus" (emphasis added). This verse may not be talking about a literal running race, but if we're going to run the race of life well, honor what God has given us, and live out our purpose—we should be as fit and healthy as we can be. We need to keep our bodies and minds healthy and in shape. We should put in the work and build physical strength. We'll be rewarded with great health and the self-esteem that comes with accepting responsibility, and we'll not only feel great, we'll look great too.

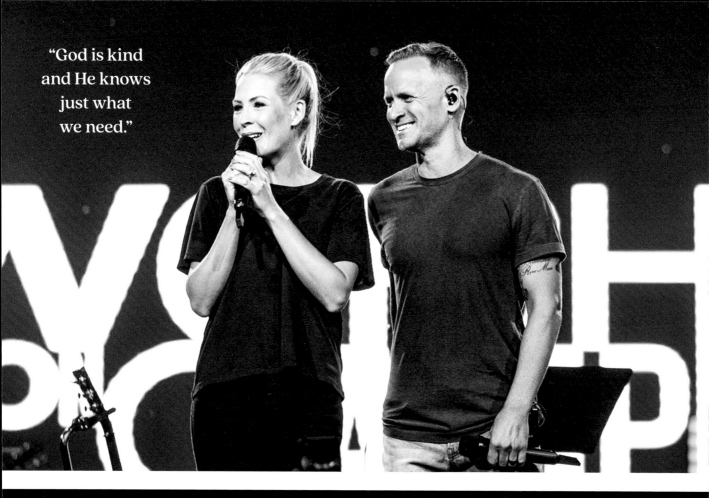

"God is kind and He knows just what we need."

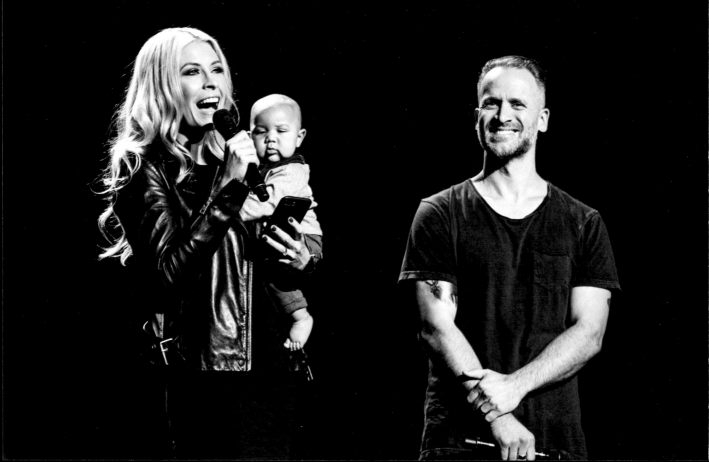

WORK, PLAY, REST

Brian and I learned a great analogy about time management years ago that has stuck with us: Picture a large glass vase. This vase symbolizes the time you have in your week. Then picture three small piles next to it: rocks, pebbles, and sand.

The rocks are the big things that must get done in your week; the pebbles matter, but less; and the sand represents things to do "if there's time left." We had to identify what the big rocks are first—the things that truly matter. Then the pebbles, and so on. **If we don't plan, the weeks will haphazardly fill with "sand" because we haven't determined what the priorities are.**

This is helpful when bringing order to your life. You need to first identify the "big rocks" of work, rest, and play—and how they are going to fit into your vase. If these are absent from your week or month, you'll experience all sorts of disconnects and stress. Instead of priorities, you'll start filling your week with sand, keeping you from the most important things in your life. That leaves you feeling like you're "all over the place." Having these three categories in healthy doses in our lives positively affects our emotions and mental health to a great degree, and, ultimately, will make or break us in the long-haul "race" of life. Instead of living chaotically or carelessly, we need to take care of ourselves holistically because it's all interconnected.

WORK

We all "work," even if the work is not defined by a résumé. Maybe we manage a company, perform surgeries, work retail, create art, or manage our households . . . it's all "work." And all work requires order and priority. Work is good for us and it's directly connected to God's purpose for our lives, but we have to watch our weaknesses, which might include laziness or overworking. (Hi, my name is Jenn Johnson, and I battle overworking.) Knowing where you're weak is half the battle.

Being a working parent has its challenges. I've definitely had "mom guilt" *many* times because I am a working mom (especially since I travel for work, often leaving the kids at home when it doesn't make sense to take them along). I've had to wrestle with hurtful comments like, "Why did you even have kids if you're gonna leave them?" (Yeah, not fun. Especially coming from someone close.) I know I was called to lead and travel, but I want to be there fully for my kids.

However, God is kind and He knows just what we need.

Around the time my mom guilt was at an all-time high, God gave me a gift. My daughter's

> "I knew I was called to be a mom, to write songs, lead teams, worship, and travel. I knew I could do it all, if I followed the Holy Spirit from season to season."

third-grade teacher at Bethel Christian School planned something special for Mother's Day every year. Instead of the kids doing a craft for their moms, she invited each mom to come in individually and the kids prayed and prophesied over each mom (not your normal school, I know—it's amazing!). I had a flight later that day for a ministry trip, but first I went in for my prayer session in my daughter's class. When I came in, I didn't tell them anything about how I was doing. I sat down in a little chair and they gathered around me and laid their hands on me. The teacher prayed and asked God to show them what He was saying about me. One by one the kids prayed and told me what they felt God was saying. In the midst of all these sweet prayers from little voices, one little boy put his hand on me and said, "You're doing a great job. And you're like a honeybee! And you have to go pollinate or this world won't be beautiful." Cue. The. Tears. That was it. That's exactly the "why" for my work and travel. God was using us not only to lead worship and write songs but to encourage and unite the global church.

Another little girl said, "And you pollinate with the love and joy of God!" More tears. The rest of what they said was a blur. I'd been struggling with accusations and mom guilt and it was exhausting. It caused me to question God's purpose for my life and I had been thrown off track. So, this little boy's image of a honeybee and pollination brought so much clarity to me. I'm thankful for teachers who train kids to hear God; kids have the same Holy Spirit an adult has. God speaks to them and uses them to change people's lives. It's beautiful. Like the Word says, "Out of the mouth of babes" (Ps. 8:2 KJV).

But here's the thing: Isn't it crazy how you can experience something so clear and personal, and then a few hours later you're questioning and swirling again? We left our kids with the grandparents and headed for the airport. On the long flight, it hit me again . . . another tidal wave of working-mom guilt came crashing down on me. Plus, I was *already* missing my kids. I tried to distract myself, watching whatever show was playing on the airplane screen, and ignore it. But I couldn't, and tears streamed down my face to the point that the flight attendant checked to see if I was okay. I sat there, sad and spaced out, waiting for the flight to end. But just then, I heard God speak to me, *Tune in to what you're watching.* Like thunder, **His voice broke me out of my fog.** I tuned in to what I had been watching for the past hour—a nature documentary on honeybees and the global benefit of cross-pollination. Um . . . what?! Are you kidding me?! I laughed out loud. "Yes, Jesus. I hear You." I knew God was smiling with this happy smirk . . . and even though it wasn't easy to be away from the kids, I was right where I was supposed to be on that plane.

I knew I was called to be a mom. I knew I was called to write songs, lead teams, worship, and travel. I knew I could do it all, *if* I followed the lead of the Holy Spirit from season to season. For me, it's meant that sometimes my work calls me away from home. And sometimes I say no to opportunities because I want to be at my kids' events or don't want to overcrowd our lives. It's a journey and a juggle, but when we follow the Holy Spirit, He guides us through it. We change, our kids change, seasons change, and we need to be pliable and willing to change, too, as God brings order and direction into our lives. Many times in my life I've just missed it completely and packed too many things into the week or month. And when that happens, all I can do is say sorry to the people in my life who are affected and try again to get it right, learning from my mistakes.

Whatever your work is today—put it on the table. Ask God about it, see if there's anything you need to get in order.

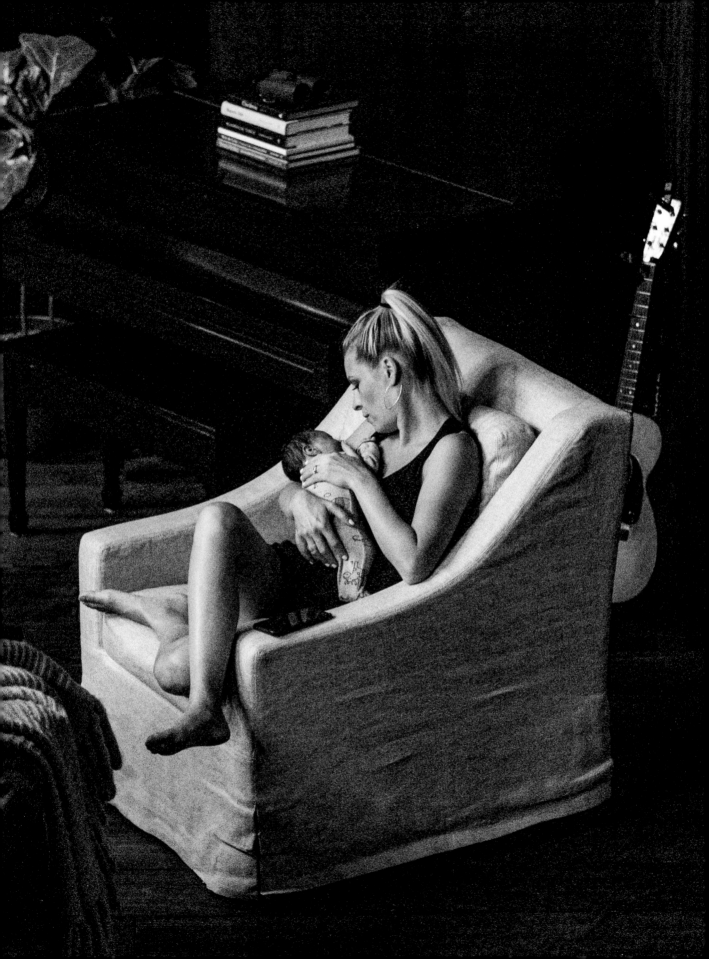

I love this verse about work:

> **Don't just do the minimum that will get you by. Do your best. Work from the heart for your real Master, for God, confident that you'll get paid in full when you come into your inheritance. Keep in mind always that the ultimate Master you're serving is Christ. The sullen servant who does shoddy work will be held responsible. Being a follower of Jesus doesn't cover up bad work.**
>
> *Colossians 3:23–25* MSG

PLAY

Whether it's hanging with friends, throwing parties, traveling, or going to an amazing restaurant . . . having fun is my favorite. It keeps us connected to people, and it's important to make sure "fun" is prioritized in our schedules. For Brian and me, it's important to have fun trips and date nights on the calendar; otherwise, the needs of the house, the kids, our friends, and work can consume us.

Whether it's socializing, traveling, reading, spending time on hobbies, or doing something new and adventurous, fun is a necessity and comes in all shapes and sizes! Play is a time when you're intentionally doing fun things. When you're doing something that *isn't* work. And it's usually something that makes you smile just thinking about it. This was difficult for me because I didn't have a hobby . . . or so I thought . . . but I found my hobby: it's adventure, hiking, and eating delicious food in beautiful spaces with Brian or friends. (Thank You, God, that Napa, California, is only a three-hour drive from us!)

Family vacations when you have little kids are

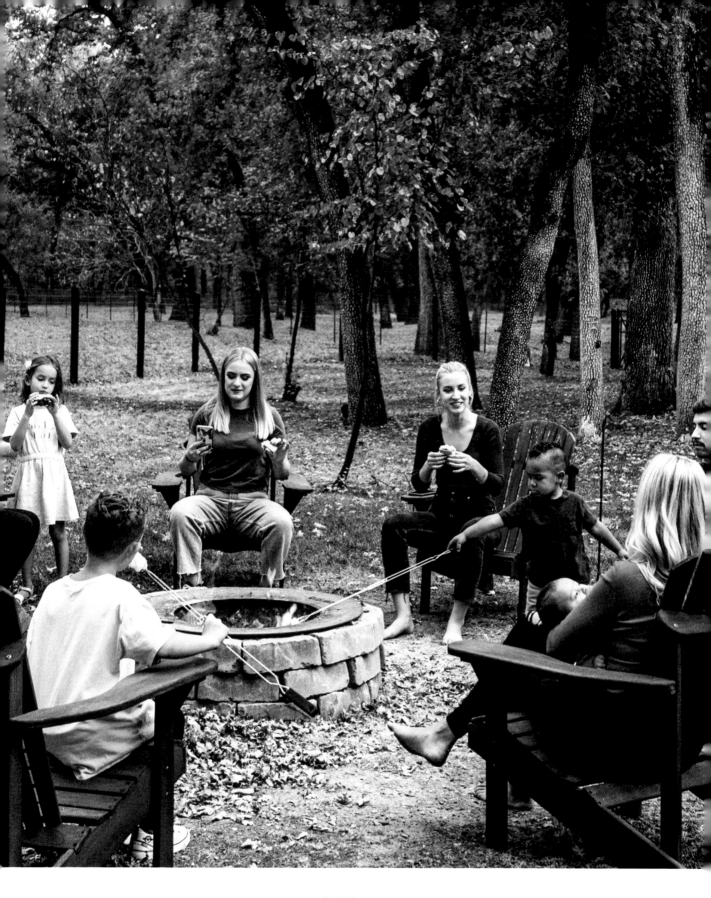

Work, Play, Rest

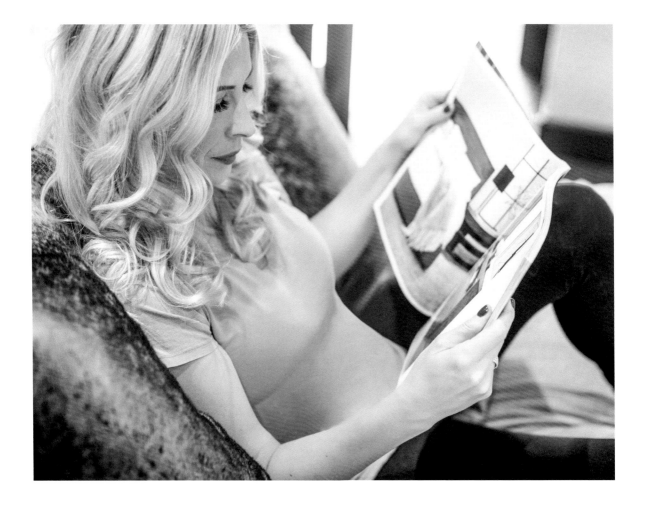

fun, but they can be exhausting. From the long travel days, hauling stuff around, making sure your toddler doesn't swallow *too* much sand, and everyone not sleeping well since they're not in their own beds . . . it's a lot. You often come home more exhausted than when you left. Brian and I got smart after a few years and budgeted to take a babysitter with us so we could have some time to ourselves on the trip. (Or you can just do a Disney cruise . . . built-in babysitting!)

Make space for play and rest—on vacations and in your everyday life—even if you have to get really creative. And it's just one more reason for having a good community around you! You can help each other by trading babysitting or sharing the things you have so others can use them (like camping gear or extra tickets to a concert or baseball game).

REST

Rest doesn't come naturally to most people, especially me. We live in a culture that glorifies busyness and hustling. We can get really caught up in the daily tasks of home, kids, friends, work, and hospitality, but if that's all we do, burnout is soon to follow. **Not resting, and being tired throughout your day as a result, will affect everything in your life!** Even if you're a lover of people and extroverted like I am, I've found it's still incredibly important for me to get alone time to rest. I have to actually say to Brian, "I need alone time" *before* I get grouchy! This took me years to figure out, but now I've seen how much better I am as a wife, mom, and friend when I've been able to rest. There are three things you can do to rest during your week:

1 | **UNWIND.** A big part of resting is finding ways to clear your mind, to unwind and relax. Some things that are restful and soul-refreshing for me include reading a home decor magazine, watching cooking shows, soaking in a magnesium bath, reading the Bible, lying in bed watching a movie, trying a new recipe, or walking alone in nature to let my mind relax. For someone else, unwinding could look like curling up with a good book, doing puzzles, drawing or painting, writing, or gardening. It could be any number of things! Find an activity that helps you rest and renew your mind, then add it to your weekly schedule, just like you would a meeting or exercise. Make rest just as prioritized and sacred as working.

2 | **RENEW YOUR MIND.** Another big part of resting is spending time in God's Word. The Word of God renews your mind and true rest is found in Him. I've found that if I neglect daily devotional time with God, I burn out and get weird *fast*. But when I start my day in His Word, even when my day is super busy and full, I find respite in His promises.

Verses to meditate on:

Truly my soul finds rest in God.

Psalm 62:1

Don't burn out; keep yourselves fueled and aflame. Be alert servants of the Master, cheerfully expectant. Don't quit in hard times; pray all the harder.

Romans 12:11–12 MSG

3 | **SLEEP.** Sounds easy, but not getting enough sleep causes a lot of problems. Whether it's the student who stays up too late and has to get up early for school or the parents of babies who wake them up throughout the night every night, many of us don't get enough sleep! Numerous studies have shown associations between not enough sleep and diabetes, obesity, hypertension, and even mortality. Sleeping a good seven to nine hours a night will benefit everything in your life, including your mood, your energy level, your health, your mind, and your patience. Just try to do the best you can to make sleep a priority. A big part of getting good sleep is having the discipline to go to bed thirty minutes before you need to be asleep so that you can wind down.

To help you sleep better, try these things:

- Minimal caffeine intake. (No caffeine after lunch is best. Want a second cup in the morning? Do decaf.)

- Take your vitamins with breakfast; otherwise, they can keep you awake at night.

- Stop eating and drinking three hours before you sleep.

- Avoid alcohol.

- Protect sleeping conditions (difficult to do with a newborn or snoring spouse, but even if you have to sleep in separate rooms . . . do it!).

- No electronics an hour before sleep. (This one is *TOUGH*!)

- Start to wind down in the evening before you actually sleep. Turn the lights down, take an Epsom salts bath, and keep your room cool.

Work, Play, Rest

Truffle Popcorn

Coconut oil

½ cup popcorn kernels

4 tablespoons butter, melted

1 tablespoon nutritional yeast

1 teaspoon dried chives

1 teaspoon fine sea salt or truffle salt

¼ teaspoon black pepper

Generously coat the bottom of a pot with coconut oil. Heat over medium-high heat until the oil is nice and hot. Add the kernels and stir until one pops. Quickly put the lid on. Grab oven mitts and stay close, giving the pan a good shake every 15 seconds so that the kernels fall to the bottom of the pan and the popcorn doesn't burn. Have a large paper bag or food container ready and the second the popcorn stops popping, dump it into the bag/container. Drizzle the melted butter onto the popcorn and shake to coat. Then sprinkle nutritional yeast, chives, salt, and pepper onto the popcorn and shake again. Eat and love your life.

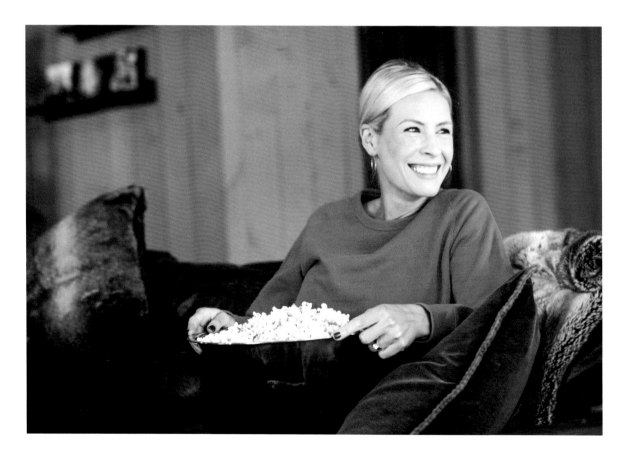

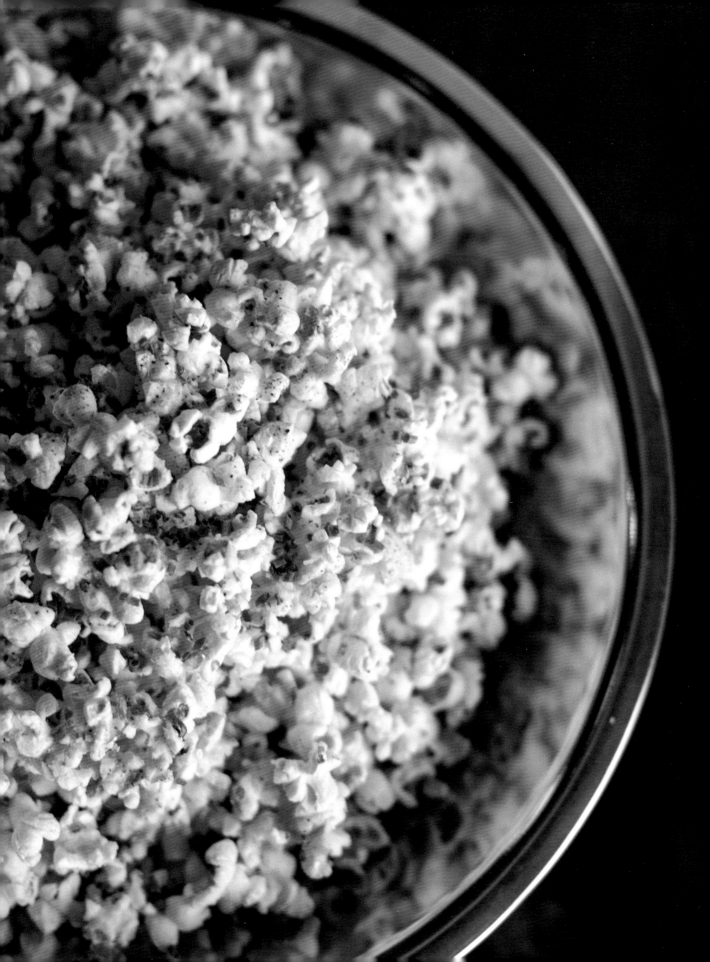

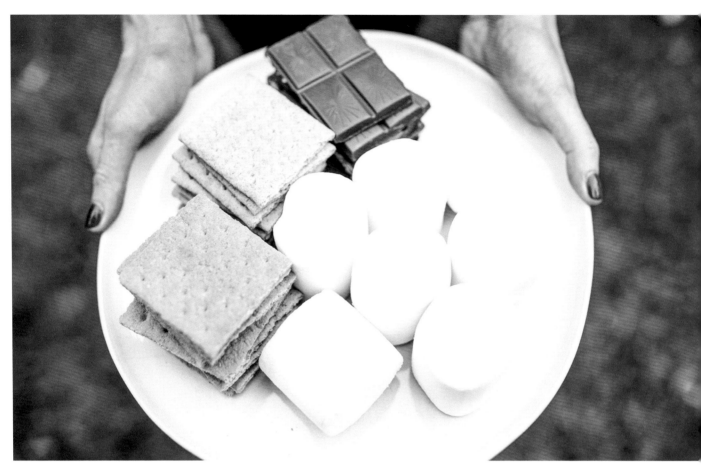

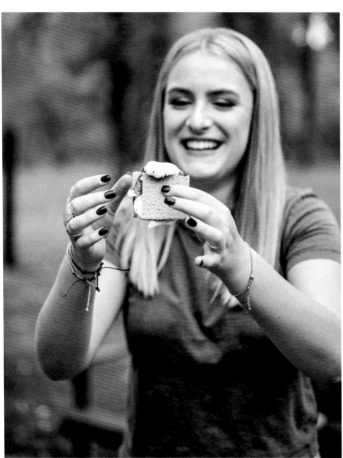

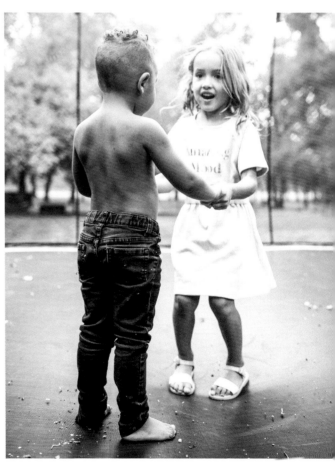

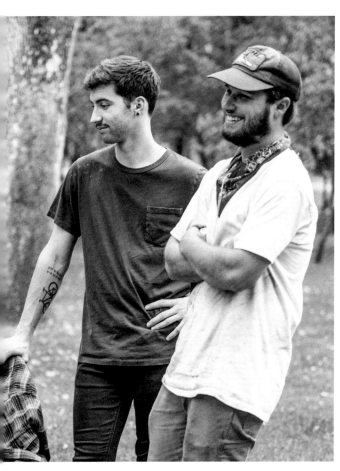

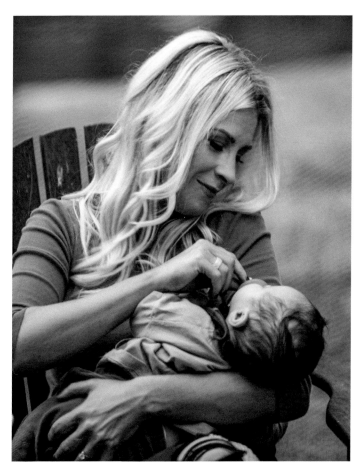

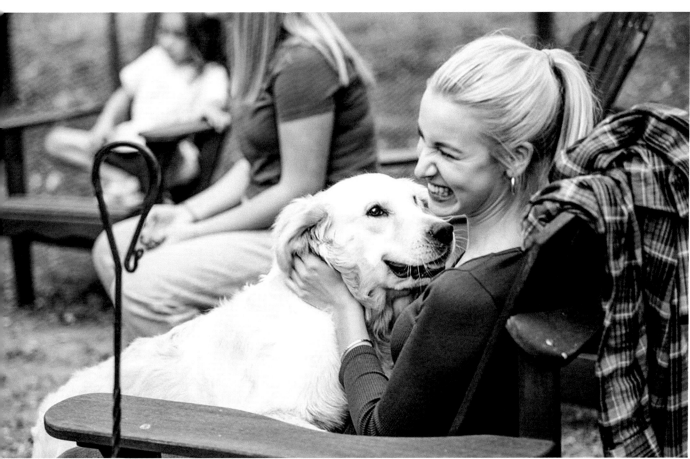

Pause and consider:

Take a minute and ask the Holy Spirit to help you identify what the "big rocks" in your life are. Do you include work, fun, and rest in your week? Use your phone or grab a pen and make a list of the things you do in your life that feel like work, rest, and fun. When you're finished, see what areas seem full or empty.

Health is a journey. From your beliefs, to what you eat, to your work-fun-rest rhythm, there is often some area of your health practices that needs attention and often more than one. Take it one step at a time. When you take care of your body—a temple of the Holy Spirit—you'll have energy to do more of the things you love and spend time with the people you love.

Since I've made major health changes in my life, I've had more energy to give my husband, kids, and friends (and I've been less grouchy); I have more energy to host; and I have more motivation to continue getting healthier in all areas of my life. It all starts with taking that next step.

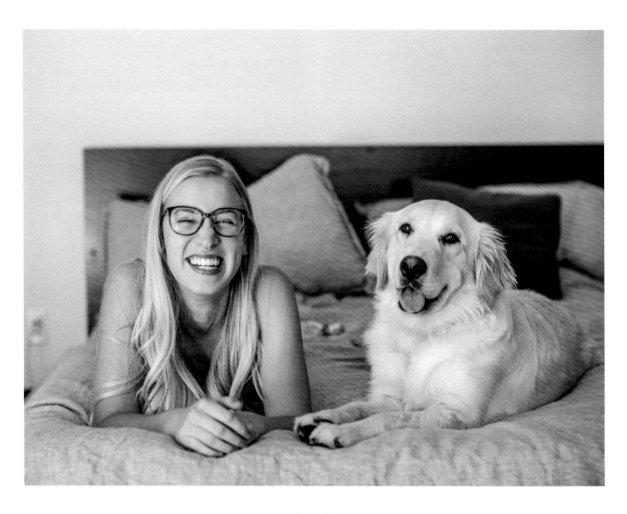

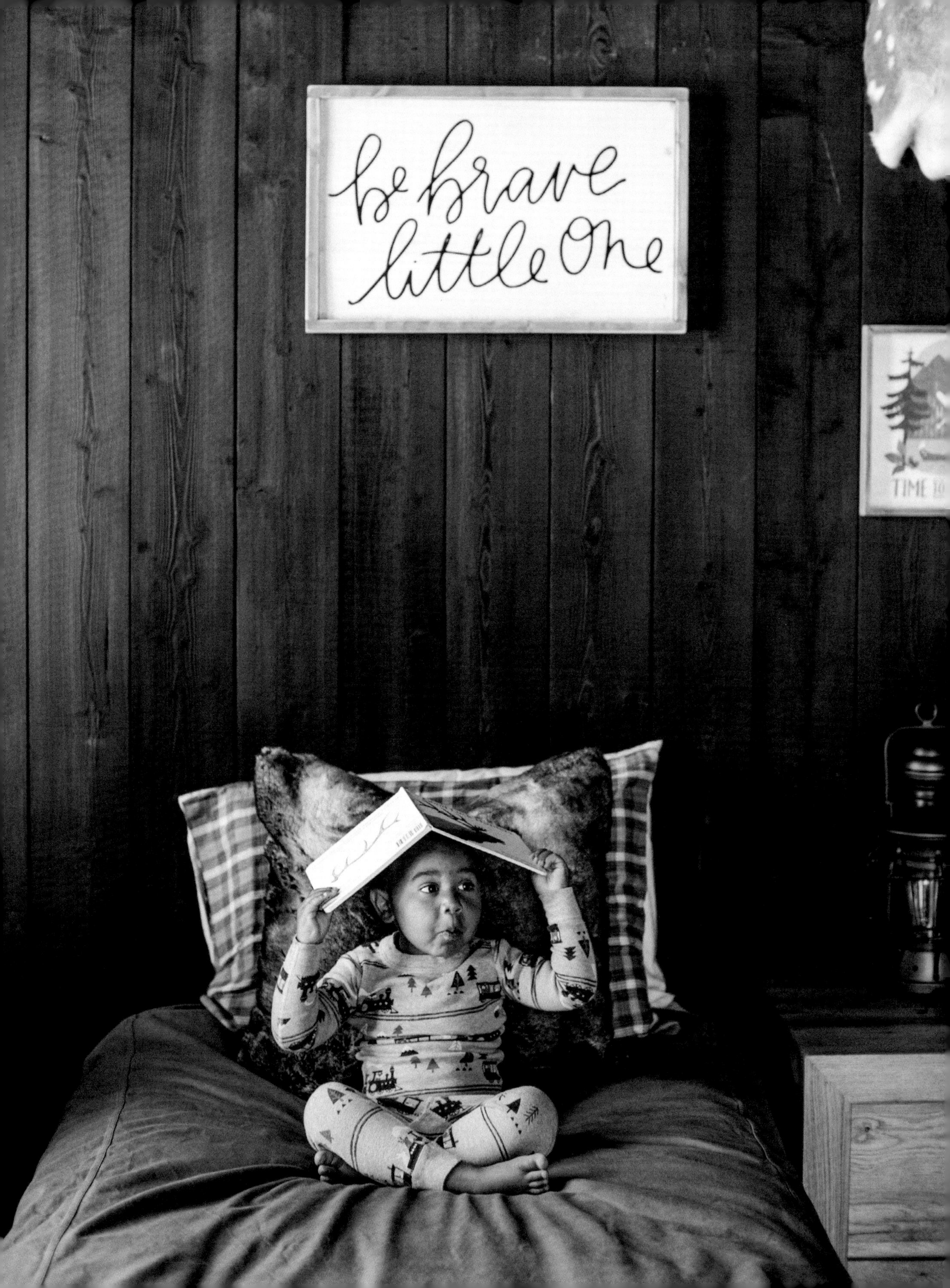
be brave
little One

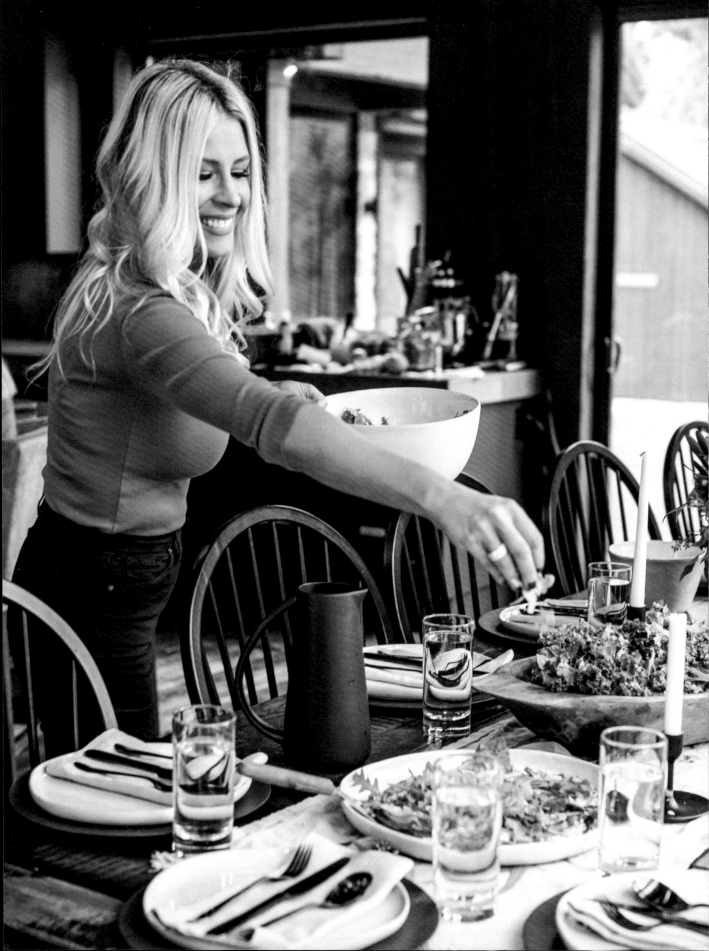

Part 04 | HOSPITALITY

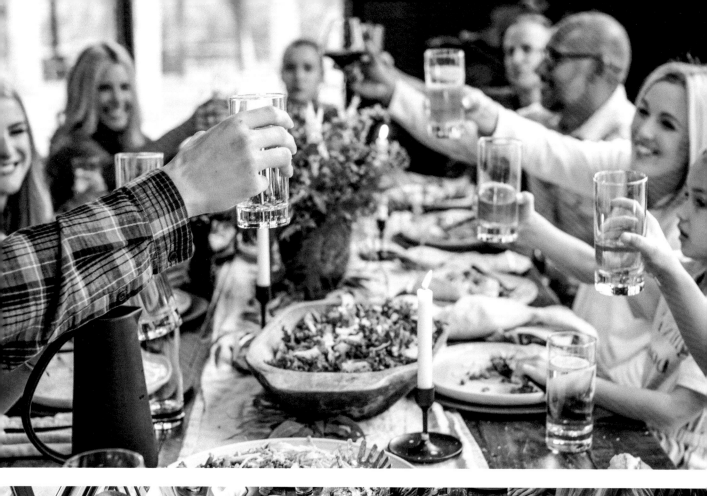
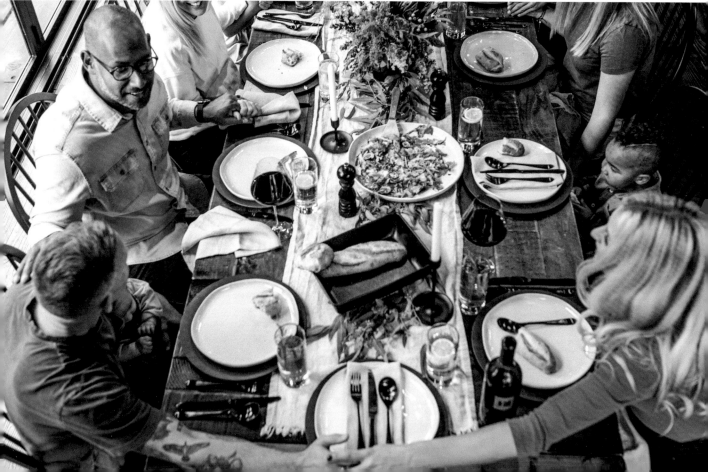

Ch. 12 | COMMUNITY

We are called to live transparently and openhandedly. When we invite God into our every moment, thought, and decision, transparency is possible.

And this will overflow into all aspects of our lives, making every relationship and community we are a part of thrive. Hospitality is all about gathering people, building community, and hosting people—sharing your lives with one another. We learn how to do this first with our family, then our friends, then our church, then people outside of the church. If you want people to experience the inviting love of God, you must first be able to invite them into your world or space.

God gives us many pictures of what strong community looks like in the Bible. From eating together, to gathering in prayer, to worshipping in every tongue, to inviting in the lost, the Scriptures give us countless examples of what biblical community is. One of my favorite examples of this is the fact that Jesus ate with people in their homes all the time. Although it seems simple, eating together is powerful! At the table we hear how people are doing. It's intimate. Happy things are shared; struggle is shared and met with care, love, and prayer. We can talk about difficult things and the connection isn't lost by trying to handle it via text. Paul says in 2 John, "I have much more to say to you, but I don't want to do it with paper and ink. For I hope to visit you soon and talk with you face to face. Then our joy will be complete" (v. 12 NLT). Being in the room with people changes everything.

Another one of my favorite examples of biblical community is in Acts 2:44–47. I love reading these verses, and all verses really, in different translations to get a more holistic understanding of the passage:

All the believers were together and had everything in common. They sold property and possessions to give to anyone who had need. Every day they continued to meet together in the temple courts. *They broke bread in their homes and ate together with glad and sincere hearts, praising God and enjoying the favor of all the people.* And the Lord added to their number daily those who were being saved. *(emphasis added)*

NIV

All the believers were in fellowship as one body, and they shared with one another whatever they had. Out of generosity they even sold their assets to distribute the proceeds to those who were in need among them. Daily they met together in the temple courts and in one another's homes to celebrate communion. They shared meals together with joyful hearts and tender

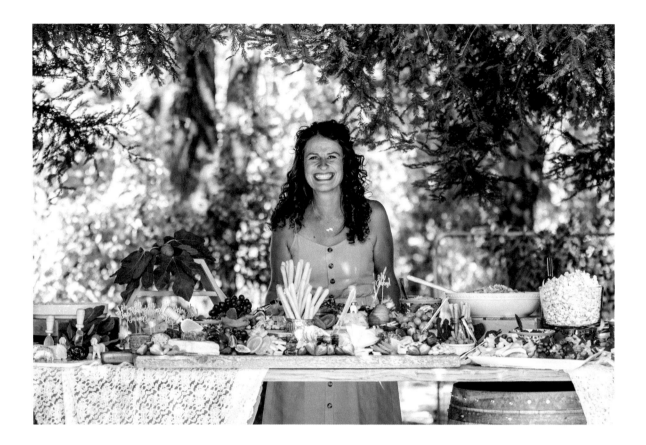

humility. They were continually filled with praises to God, enjoying the favor of all the people. And the Lord kept adding to their number daily those who were coming to life.

TPT

All the believers were together and had everything in common. Selling their possessions and goods, they shared with anyone who was in need. With one accord they continued to meet daily in the temple courts and to break bread from house to house, sharing their meals with gladness and sincerity of heart, praising God and enjoying the favor of all the people. And the Lord added to their number daily those who were being saved.

BSB

It's so inspiring! And such a practical guide to what hospitality in community looks like:

- Be generous.
- Gather and eat together.
- Praise God.
- Enjoy the favor.
- Get people saved.

Building community is being there for one another. I love this passage from Hebrews:

And let us consider how to stir up one another to love and good works, not neglecting to *meet together*, as is the habit of some, but *encouraging one another*, and all the more as you see the Day drawing near.

10:24–25 ESV, emphasis added

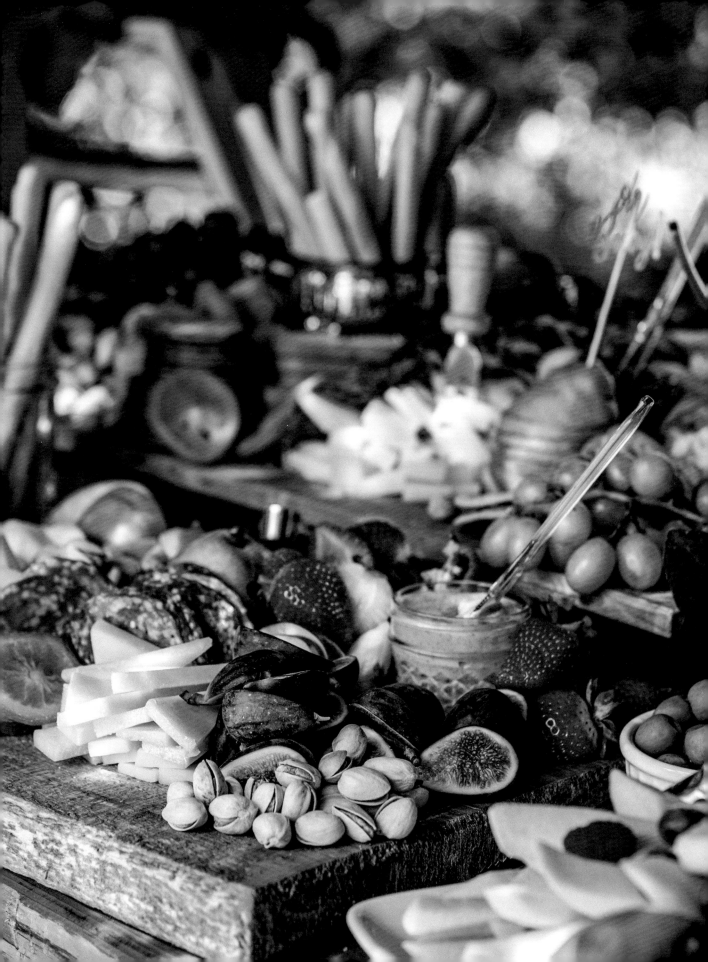

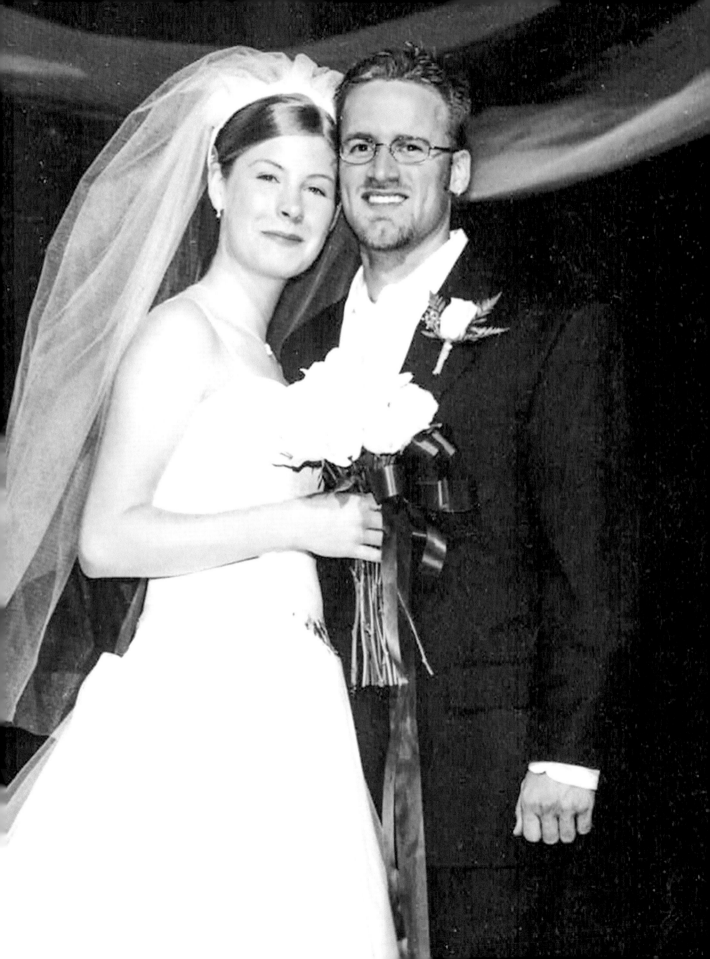

Growing up in a small town and attending a small church, I saw firsthand the beauty of the church community and the spirit of hospitality very present in it: Christ-centered believers who loved and cared for one another and reached out to those who didn't yet know Jesus and loved them well. From potlucks to wedding showers to bringing meals to someone who'd just had a baby, the church was so much more than people who attended a weekly service. The church was about the Father's business (see Luke 2:49), for His kingdom to come. I knew from a young age that I wanted to be involved in the church, leading people to Christ. I wanted to get married and have a family that was rooted in God, and I wanted our home to be a gathering space for all people, from every background, to come to know, love, and worship God. I wanted a husband who had the same heart, and I found him . . . Brian Johnson.

I first met Brian when I was about twelve . . . at church camp. (Don't write off those camp crushes!) Brian was sixteen, super cute, and probably didn't know I existed. I remember watching him play football (swoon) from the cabin porch while eating sunflower seeds with his sister Leah. Brian's dad, Bill, preached and led worship at our camps and church meetings, and many times his whole family would come.

Over the years, Leah and I became friends, hanging out after meetings and at camp.

When I was seventeen, my family and I moved to Redding, and I started hanging out with Leah at the Johnsons' house. Seeing that I wasn't twelve anymore, Brian noticed me. Needless to say, many girls liked him. He was the single, quiet, cute worship leader who was pursuing God in ministry school. I didn't want to be one of the girls at the front of the stage while he was leading, so I would go to the back of the sanctuary during worship. I couldn't stop thinking about him, though. I was in the prayer chapel on our church's property one day praying and worshipping and I said, "God, I moved

here to focus on YOU. Not him. Either I'm marrying him or take these feelings away! Yes or no, am I marrying him?" No answer. God probably rolled His eyes and laughed at me.

But then, as I walked out of the prayer house toward the main campus building, Brian walked up to me. He said, "Can I talk to you in my office?"

"Um, yes," I responded, trying not to smile too big and thinking to myself, *You can talk to me for the rest of your life if you want!* We sat down in his office and he started by saying, "I really like you." The rest is really a blur, but I remember that he talked about this connection he felt we had, what he saw in me, and then he asked me what I thought. I was shocked. Excited, *so* happy . . . and shocked. I told him what I'd been praying only a few minutes before, and then . . . this. We both sat there and smiled. "So we're dating?" he said. I nodded and smiled, and that was that . . . we were dating.

Our first week together was amazing. We felt we were more than just dating, and really on the journey toward engagement, however crazy that sounded or felt. We felt like we had known each other our whole lives, and being together just felt . . . natural and right.

After we had been dating for ten days (yes . . . ten days), we were together onstage. I was playing keyboard and Brian was about to start leading worship for the Sunday night service at church. Brian started to play and then prayed over the mic, "Let's just start to stir ourselves up for the Lord . . ." Eyes closed and hands raised, I prayed along. Then, over the mic, he said, "One more thing before we start worship. Jenn . . . will you marry me?" as he pulled a ring out of his pocket. The crowd *literally* went wild. I opened my eyes and looked over at him, wide-eyed with the biggest smile, nodding as I walked toward him. I had no idea he would propose so soon.

He had already met with my parents and received their blessing . . . a true miracle. Even though it was unconventional, and I was seventeen

Community

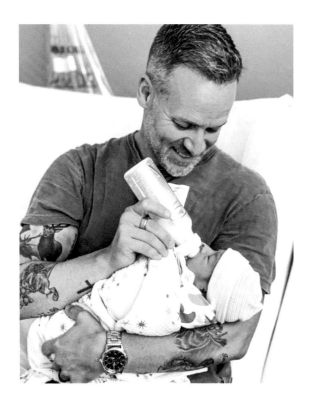
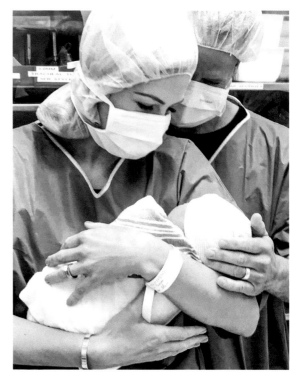

(yes . . . seventeen), they felt God was moving in our lives and his parents did as well. It didn't make any sense (following the Holy Spirit doesn't many times), but it was perfect! He put the ring on my finger, we kissed, and then went straight into worship with stupid, huge smiles on our faces. That was that, and seven months later (after a lot of great marriage counseling and inner healing), I got married to my summer camp crush.

We had an amazing first year of marriage even though we had plenty of "bumps in the road" as both of us grew in new ways. On our one-year anniversary, we were away on vacation and found out we were pregnant! We were SO excited, as were our families. And eight months later, our first baby girl, Haley Bren, was born. Life was good. Other than learning to be parents, our life was a lot of leading worship, giving piano lessons, pastoring, writing, recording, house renovation, and me learning to cook more dishes. A few years later, our second baby girl, Tèa Kate, was born. And a few years after that, our first son, Braden Tyler, was born. We loved watching our

family grow and our kids' little personalities start to show as we taught them about life and God.

When Brian and I first got married, we talked about how we would love to have biological children and that we were also open to adoption if God ever laid that on our hearts. Seventeen years of being married and three biological children later, we thought we were done, but God spoke to us in 2017 while we were watching a TV show where a family had adopted a child. We sat there holding each other and the presence of God filled the room. I looked up at Brian and said, "I'd do it." And he instantly responded, "I would too." I was shocked! I couldn't believe those words were coming out of his mouth and I don't think he could either! Our youngest at the time was ten years old. We had been out of diapers for eight years. Were we *really* saying we would go back to that? This was *crazy*, but **we both knew it: God had another baby for us and we were to adopt.** We prayed that night for more confirmation, and God spoke to us both in different verses in the Bible. Mine was James 1:27: "Religion

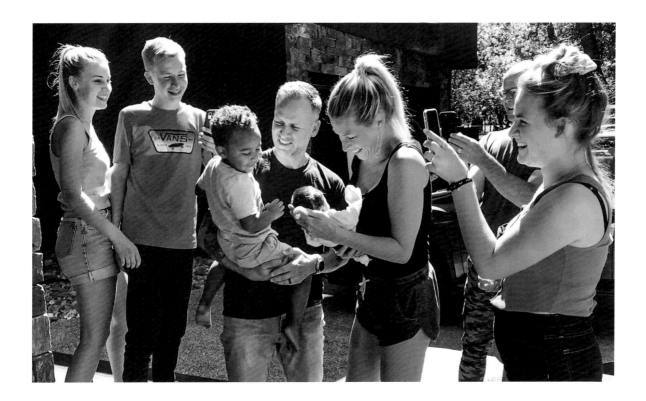

that God our Father accepts as pure and faultless is this: to look after orphans and widows in their distress and to keep oneself from being polluted by the world." (This is an incredible charge to Christians to ask God how we can care for orphans and widows personally.)

We sat our three kids down the next day and told them we had something to tell them. (We secretly filmed it, too, and it's an epic video of laughter, screams of excitement, and tears of joy.) Needless to say . . . they were elated. Our middle daughter said she had prayed every night for years for this. We were all in. We knew we were to adopt a newborn boy, so we and our kids began to dream of a name. I don't remember whose idea it was first, but we all landed on the perfect name for our new little buddy . . . Ryder Moses, meaning "Messenger. Deliverer." Yep. That was it.

The next day we jumped into the process. Paperwork, fingerprinting, all of it. It was a quick process, nothing short of supernatural, and we got matched a few months later. Our son was born just

weeks after that and we got to be in the room. It was a holy moment. They placed Ryder Moses in our arms, and it was an *instant* bond . . . Our hearts melted. We had been praying for him and his birth mom since we first felt we were to adopt. And she was incredible; talk about courage: to know that you can't emotionally care for a child but yet have the courage to carry, give birth to, and choose a family to parent your child.

Ryder Moses is the greatest. We don't know what we would do without him. He is such a joy and gift to our whole family. And he's adorable, with his beautiful brown skin, gorgeous eyes, and cheeky smile.

We thought we might be done after that, but nope, God spoke to us to **adopt** *again* in 2020. We jumped in headfirst, one more time and with a very similar process, and our son Malachi Judah was born and came into our home. People ask us now if we will adopt again and my answer is, only God knows! But **if God told us to, we would for sure do it**, and these two wonderful little boys are SO loved by us, our oldest three, our extended families, and our community.

Our families have taught us much about what it means to be in community, and God has further grown that concept for us. Not the bless-your-heart, see-you-at-the-next-potluck kind of community, but the kind of community where they know all your junk, love you anyway, encourage you, and call you higher in love. When you're building this kind of community, it's important to ask God who your "circle" of people are, and then see the people in your circle in this way. Commit to go deeper than the surface with them, to be "in their corner" in return . . . all in . . . emotionally, physically, and spiritually (holistically).

We need people in our lives who keep us healthy and focused on Jesus, who give us life and who are there with us through thick and thin, to celebrate the highs of life and grieve the lows. These deep connections to other people are what we're designed to experience—how we're wired. This is what God has for all of us. And it's why relationships are a priority in my life.

But good, healthy relationships don't just "happen." You have to plant and grow them by paying attention to who's around you and then putting time and energy toward connecting and growing those relationships.

Whether I'm looking at my own relationships or helping others sort through theirs, I like to break them down into three categories:

1| People **you're closest to**.

2| People **who are leading you**.

3| People **you are leading**.

Often, it's only the first category—close friends—that gets the most attention for what a good community is supposed to look like. People imagine that if they have "close friends" in their lives, they're all set. Yes, those people are critical, but it's the combination of all three categories that really brings health and wholeness. If you don't have all three, you're likely experiencing gaps in your life. Or if you have all three categories filled,

but it's not with people who are pushing you in the right direction, "as iron sharpens iron" friends (see Prov. 27:17), you can go downhill fast. I've heard it said that **"you become like the people you hang out with,"** and that is very true.

PEOPLE YOU'RE CLOSEST TO

It's one thing to be friendly to everyone, but this is about who's in your inner circle. You need "through thick and thin" people who speak into your life, as you speak into theirs. Let God lead you into divine friendships and sometimes *out* of friendships that you shouldn't be in. You don't necessarily have to stop being friends with someone, but who you keep closest to you matters, and this can change. God will bring you the people you need, people who love you and are committed to your growth and maturity as a Christian, but it will take effort to plant and grow those relationships. **Just ask Him to show you "who and how." Don't alienate yourself. The sheep that isn't part of the flock gets picked off by the wolf.** Good, healthy community is out there for you. Ask the Holy Spirit to lead you to those people.

One of my through-thick-and-thin friends is Heather Diane Armstrong. She and her family moved to Redding around 2006, and we became instant best friends. Heather is the most thoughtful, warmhearted, lovingly evangelistic person ever; and, she's an *incredible* photographer. (She took most of the pictures in this book!)

We've been through a LOT together with marriage, ministry, work, and kids. She is such a gift. She listens to the Holy Spirit and is sensitive to obey whatever He tells her to do. We make sure we have time together every week to either get our nails done, go for a walk, or watch our favorite shows together, and thankfully our husbands love each other so we do a lot of double dates. Heather is someone I can have fun with, be real with, and also share the highs and lows of life with. I don't know what I'd do without her!

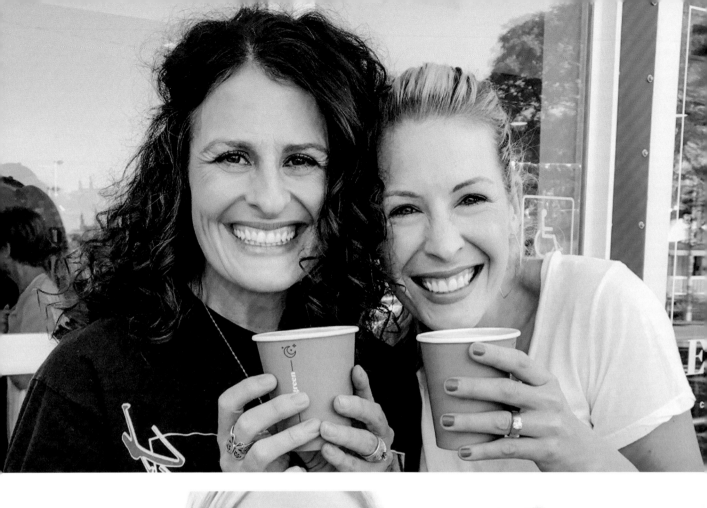
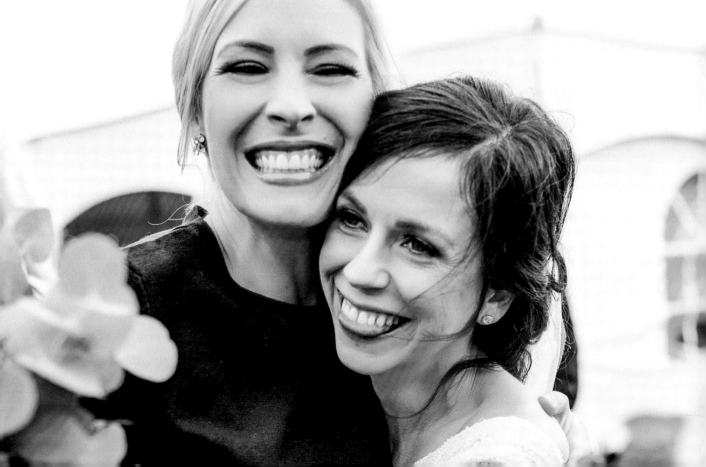

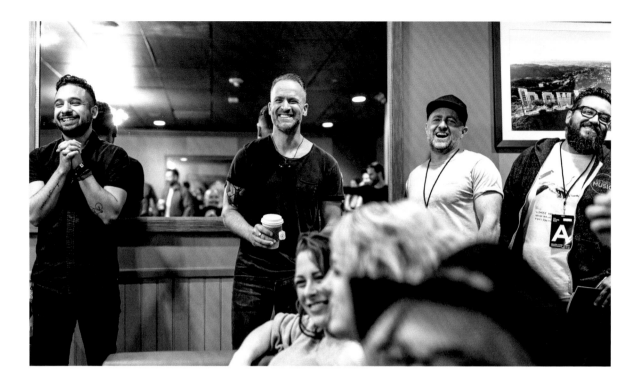

Sometimes you and your close friends will go through devastating times, which is all the more reason why you need your inner circle to be Holy Spirit–filled and healthy so they inspire you and pull you "up" in life—not drag you down. As much as we celebrate and laugh with our close friends, we also go through some serious life in the trenches with them. Death, divorce, affairs, loss, natural disasters, abuse . . . Life is intense, but the power of friendship and community is a reinforcement for our hearts, just like the way our community was there for me during Brian's nervous breakdown, refusing to let me sink. Community rallies together, prays together, holds one another up, and worships together. From bringing dinner over to babysitting, they're aware of one another's needs and love deeply.

When grief hits like a freight train, the power of God and community helps us to stay standing . . . our faith stays strong even though our flesh is weak. Just like a redwood forest does in a storm, roots deep in the ground, interconnected, relying on one another's strength to withstand the storm. Together.

I am so grateful to God for these friendships that make up our community. I can't imagine how we'd have gotten through that time without our circle coming around us: friends who prayed and worshipped over Brian through the night, friends who brought us meals and gave us verses God was showing them . . . they didn't let us go through it alone. We were surrounded. And now that we've made it through that intense season of our lives, it makes celebrations and gatherings with our community even sweeter. No matter what we go through or even the tension and the struggle that come with friendship sometimes, we all mean a lot to one another, and that will never change.

PEOPLE WHO ARE LEADING YOU

Having people who will speak honestly into your life, and challenge you toward health and wholeness, are *vital*. We all need this! It keeps us from getting tunnel vision, helps us to avoid blind spots, and gives us good shoulders to stand on.

For both Brian and me, our parents are some of those people leading us. I remember years ago, we were riding in the car with Brian's dad in Nashville to an event. Brian and I were going to lead worship and Bill would be preaching. We'd had a crazy day of travel delays, our kids were with us (and they were sick, which is like parenting a baby T. rex), and we barely made it to the car on time that day. I was in a *mood*. Trying to get myself ready to worship and change the gears of my attitude, I quietly muttered, "Mommy hat off. Worship hat on." Just barely audible. Well, it turns out that it was audible enough for my father-in-law to hear. Bill leaned over and said kindly, "The problem is . . . the 'worship hat' should have never come off."

Shot to the heart.

He got me. I closed my eyes, took a deep breath, and let it out slowly. "Right," I said back.

That one phrase changed my life. Worship isn't just music or words . . . worship is every aspect of your life: it's your heart, your attitude, your life when no one's watching . . . whatever you're doing . . . as an offering to God. So whether you're changing diapers or singing on a stage or choosing what show to watch . . . it's all worship.

> Take your everyday, ordinary life—your sleeping, eating, going-to-work, and walking-around life—and place it before God as an offering.
>
> *Romans 12:1–2* MSG

When you have people leading you, you **get checked and held accountable to higher standards**. And **you do want this**, even if it's hard to hear the truth sometimes! We are called to help one another be better, and that means inviting people into our lives who have our permission to do that. Be purposeful in finding this accountability. Find people you feel God is highlighting to you. Ask them if they would pray about being one of your iron-sharpens-iron people. If they say yes, ask them to let you know of any encouragement they have for you or ways they see in which you need to grow.

PEOPLE YOU'RE LEADING

No matter what name you give it—discipleship, mentoring, coaching, managing, parenting—this part of community has big value for both you and the ones you're leading. If you're leading someone well, you are kept in a place that's accountable. Someone is looking to you, so you are more likely to live by good example. Leadership also challenges and refines you, because you want to pass along all the wisdom and helpful advice you can.

Titus 1:7–9 is an amazing guide for how we should behave as leaders:

> Since an overseer manages God's household, he must be blameless—not overbearing, not quick-tempered, not given to drunkenness, not violent, not pursuing dishonest gain. Rather, **he must be hospitable, one who loves what is good, who is self-controlled, upright, holy and disciplined.** He must hold firmly to the trustworthy message as it has been taught, so that he can encourage others by sound doctrine and refute those who oppose it. *(emphasis added)*

One thing I've found to be useful when leading others and encouraging them toward health and Jesus is to pay attention and ask questions. When you're discerning that something seems "off" in a person's life, even if you don't have anything more than instinct, ask questions about it: "How's this going?" "What's your relationship with this person like?" "This makes me nervous . . . Talk to me about it."

I found this approach to be helpful with a member of our community whom we're close to and leading. I could sense something was unhealthy—not overtly, but somewhere in the background. I didn't go to the person finger-pointing—that's never a good idea! I just started the conversation with, "I love you, so that's why we're here. What's going on? You doing okay?" The floodgates opened. They hadn't even realized that something was off, because it was still subtle and nothing obviously sinful, but in that conversation it was like God started weeding through this person's heart and showing us what needed to change. When we love each other well, we aren't only encouraging, we are calling each other out on our junk. Talking through difficult situations is best handled face-to-face. In a world of technology, we can miss an opportunity to connect by instead sending a text or an email. I highly advise sitting down with someone to talk in person when dealing with difficult situations, especially correction.

Pause and consider:

1 | **Someone you're close to**
Make a list of the people in your inner circle, your best friends, your go-to people. Look at your list and think about these questions: Does the list represent a solid community of close friends? Is there anything missing? Is there anyone on the list who might be taking up unhealthy space in your life?

2 | **Someone who's leading you**
Write down the name of anyone who is leading you—people you actually take advice from and let that advice affect your behavior or beliefs. What was the last thing you remember changing in your life because of a leader's voice? If you have leaders but they're not speaking into your real-life behaviors, have you invited them to do that? How could you approach them to start doing that?

3 | **Someone you're leading**
Who's the person or people you're leading? Make a list. Next to the name, write down a few notes about how you're leading them and any questions you might need to be asking as you pay attention to their lives. Also, if you've been a Christian for even a minute, congratulations! You're a leader; you're called to lead people to Jesus.

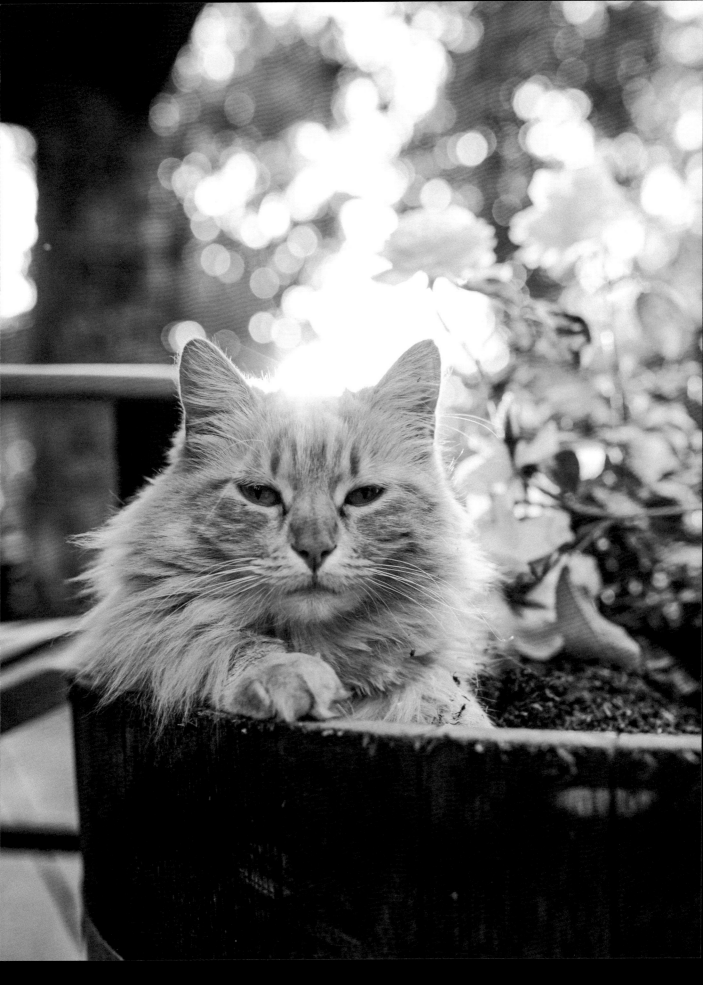

Kale Salad

6 cups kale, stems removed

⅓ cup fresh lemon juice

1 teaspoon salt

½ teaspoon black pepper

1½ cups extra-virgin olive oil

4 garlic cloves, peeled and finely minced

2 cups sliced almonds or toasted pumpkin seeds

1½ cups freshly grated Parmesan cheese

Tear the kale leaves and wash them thoroughly in cold water. Dry the leaves, then put them in a large bowl and set aside.

In a small container with a lid (I use a mason jar), combine the lemon juice, salt, and pepper. Slowly whisk in the olive oil and garlic.

Pour the dressing over the kale and use your hands or salad tongs to evenly distribute the dressing. Cover and place in the refrigerator for about 20 minutes so the dressing softens the kale.

When you take the salad out of the fridge, sprinkle with the sliced almonds or toasted pumpkin seeds, freshly grated Parmesan, and salt and pepper to taste.

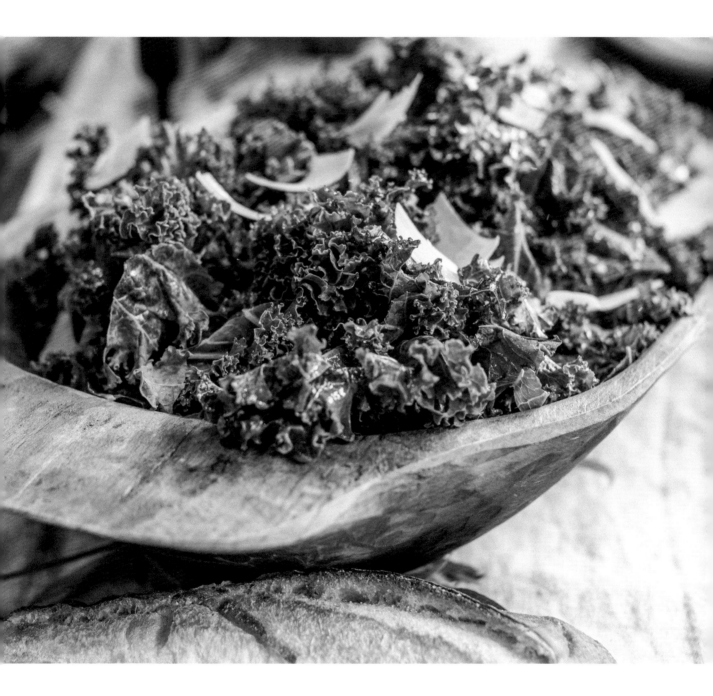

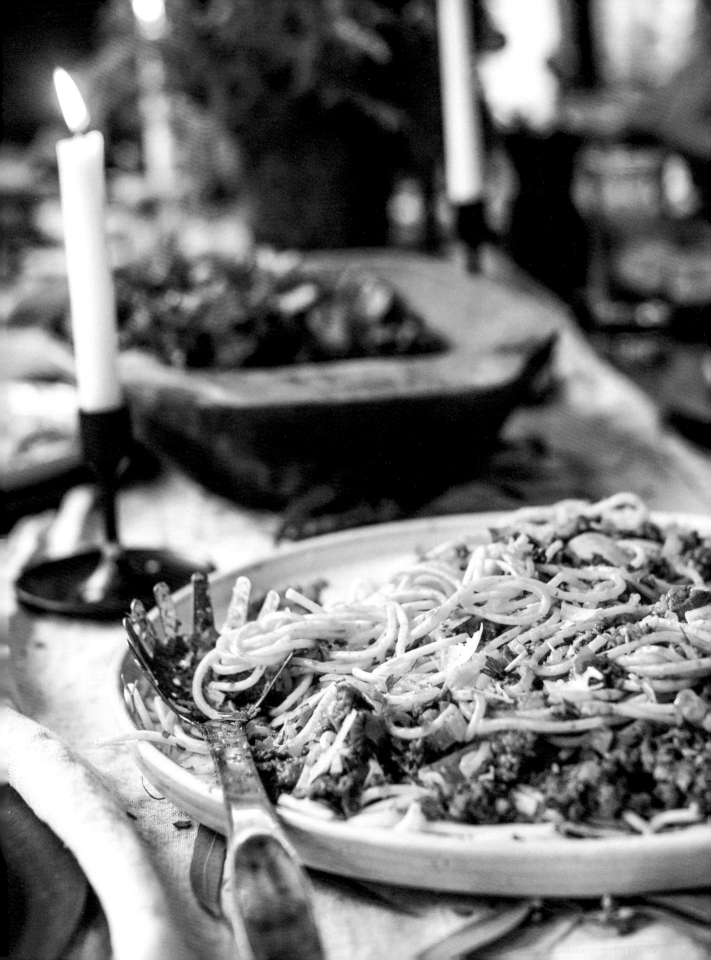

Pasta Bolognese

5 tablespoons extra-virgin olive oil

1 tablespoon butter

⅔ cup finely diced onion

⅔ cup finely diced baby carrots

⅔ cup finely diced celery

2 ounces pancetta, finely diced

½ pound extra-lean ground beef

½ pound ground pork

2 teaspoons minced garlic

½ cup finely diced mushrooms

¾ cup dry white wine

1 (28-ounce) can peeled San Marzano tomatoes, blended

1 cup chicken broth

½ teaspoon dried thyme

1 bay leaf

Salt and freshly ground black pepper

¼ cup heavy cream

2 pounds of your favorite pasta or zucchini noodles

Freshly grated Parmesan and fresh thyme (for serving)

Add 1 tablespoon olive oil and 1 tablespoon butter to a large saucepan over medium-high heat; heat until simmering. Add the onion, carrot, celery, and pancetta. Cook, stirring occasionally, until the vegetables are softened (about 7 to 8 minutes). Remove and set aside.

Next, add 4 tablespoons of olive oil to the saucepan and heat until the mixture starts to simmer. Add the ground beef and pork and cook over medium-high until almost cooked through, about 5 minutes. Return the vegetable mixture to the saucepan. Add the garlic and mushrooms and cook another 1 to 2 minutes.

Add the wine, stirring occasionally, until it has almost evaporated. Stir in the tomatoes, chicken broth, thyme, and bay leaf. Season with a generous amount of salt and pepper and bring to a boil over high heat. Cover partially and cook over medium-low heat for 1 hour, stirring occasionally. Take out the bay leaf. Stir in the heavy cream and cook the sauce until it's hot again. (You can leave out the heavy cream for a healthier option.)

Then, in a large pot of generously salted boiling water, cook the pasta until al dente. Drain the pasta and pour the sauce into the pot. Return the pasta to the pot and toss with the sauce. Serve with Parmesan and thyme sprinkled on top.

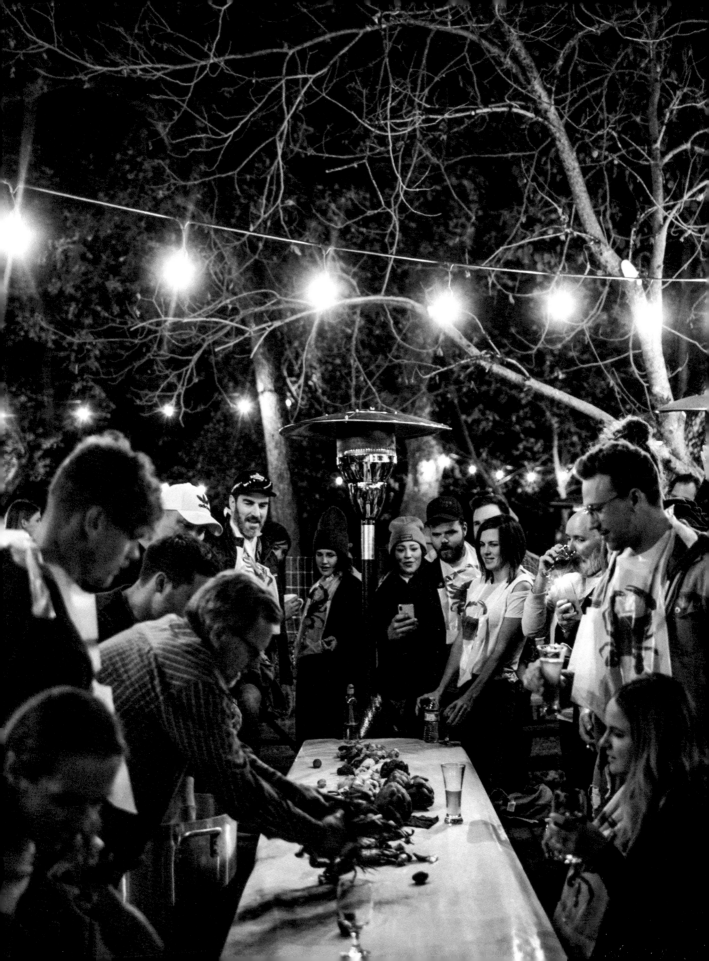

Ch. 13 | GATHERING

From sanctuaries to theaters, homes, or anyplace else where "two or more are gathered" (Matt. 18:20 KJV), THIS is the church.

From the small group of believers described in the "upper room" encounter of Acts 2, to the local church where anyone can come, we need space and time for our tight-knit circle and also for inviting in new people.

Everyone needs community. Most people are just waiting for an invite. Many people are trying to find their place to fit in. Notice the people you're surrounded by and ask God to show you who you should gather. Invite diversity into your home. Every party doesn't need to be the same group of friends or the "expected" combination. What happens when you gather diverse groups to celebrate each other is nothing short of supernatural. Brian and I love to connect people who might not otherwise cross paths to celebrate what God is doing through all of them . . . and to celebrate what He's doing around the world! We don't all believe exactly the same, but *what unites us is by far greater than anything we might disagree on.* From ethnicity to denomination, God beautifully displays **the body of Christ in diversity.** Not one church or movement "has it all." We need one another! And **we see the fullness of His beauty in each other.**

In your gatherings, open the conversation to people from unique backgrounds and people who don't normally end up sitting across the table from each other. Watch for those God is highlighting. Connect with them! I have invited people over that I just met because I felt a connection, and many of them are my closest friends to this day. Some of them had just moved here and didn't know anyone. People are looking for community. You may be the answer to their prayers. I love to invite someone new to my girlfriends' brunch and introduce them to everyone. And remember, a great line to start a conversation with is: "Tell me about you." Helping new people to feel included and like family is so important.

We host gathering after gathering at our house to build community and connect people. We always wanted our home to be a gathering space for people, and we built it with intentionality to create a warm, open, and inviting space for people to come and feel "at home." We know the reward, and it's a beautiful thing. The kingdom—the church—is meant to be a thriving, diverse, and joyful community. People who love God show they care by meeting together and encouraging one another (see Heb. 10:25).

One of the ways we have done that is by simply creating a space for people to hang out. With five kids and their friends, our own friends, our team, and the people who help us run the zoo that is our life, it's a revolving door at our house and we love it. We have soooo many people over on a weekly basis.

We encourage our kids to have their friends over whenever they want and we try to have our home be a place that kids can come and feel loved. We keep the kitchen stocked with snacks and sparkling water and we keep pizza-making ingredients at the ready. Our heart is that people can feel at "home" and part of our family in the space we've created.

From hosting baby showers, birthday parties, girlfriends' brunch, local worship community nights, global leader gatherings, youth connect groups, and everything in between, it's beautiful to watch what happens when you have no agenda but to love people, feed them great food, and celebrate diversity. **This kind of intentionality is the heart of hospitality.**

Shortly after Brian and I got married, we were handed the leadership of the Bethel Church Worship Team in Redding, California. I was eighteen and Brian was twenty-two. Overnight we became the leaders of a worship team whose members were of every age, skill, ability, and personality you could imagine. We were supposed to be leading people, some of whom were decades older than us, including *both* of Brian's grandfathers, some of his cousins, a sibling, and an aunt who had been in charge of the whole thing before they turned it over to us. It was a rough season and there were some serious low points, no doubt about it. We had a vision for the team, but it was going to take work. We had a high value for the Word of God, the presence of God, freedom, excellence, hard work, integrity, and following the Holy Spirit.

Some of the worship team left the church because they were offended by us and our new direction. But we had taken this role and we were committed to the vision God had given us; we were going to stay true to that even if it was unpopular. We wanted the church to experience God as they worshipped and not be distracted by chaos. And, we wanted to be honest with our team. It was messy, but when you remodel anything, you have to tear things down to build something new. It doesn't mean the old version was bad, just that the vision God was leading us in was . . . different.

The verse I held on to for comfort was this:

Behold, I am doing a new thing.

Isaiah 43:19 ESV

The worship team restoration took years, teaching people how to play together, not to play over one another, and to follow the Holy Spirit. And then there were all the other moving parts like figuring out how to fine-tune the sound, invest in the right equipment and sound engineer, and plan the worship set lists while still allowing the Holy Spirit to lead us in what to play and when to play it. After we got through the worship team renovation, the team started to grow as people joined the team because they loved the vision. We were practicing once a week in the evening but could see we needed more time together. We needed community, and to really get to know one another. Because it's one thing to be on a worship team, but it's entirely different when you know the other members personally and the gifts God has given them. Time spent connecting with people helps you learn their strengths *and* their weaknesses, so you can work well together, help each other, and truly love the people on your team.

We ditched our weekly evening practice and decided to have three-hour sound checks before each worship set so the band could rehearse. We also started having "worship community nights"—cramming the team into our family's great room or backyard so we could spend time together eating, worshipping, listening to each other's needs and testimonies, and praying for each other. We stayed sensitive to what God was speaking and would often ask someone from the team, church staff, or a guest to share. It was my favorite time: God, community, food, the church. We were there for one another and there to serve the church, locally and globally.

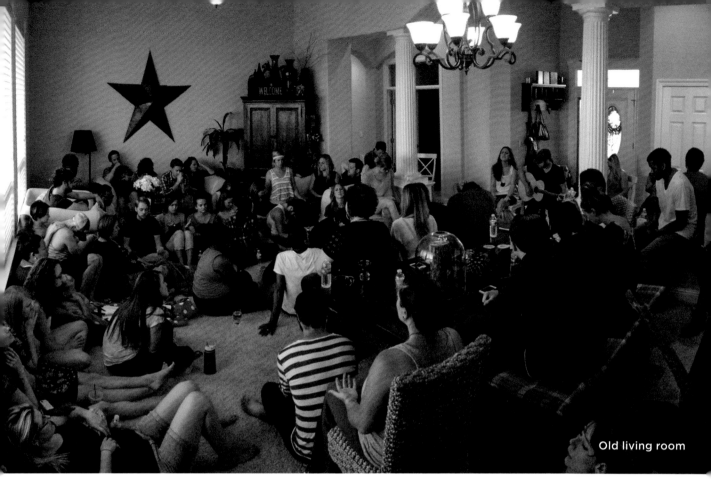

Old living room

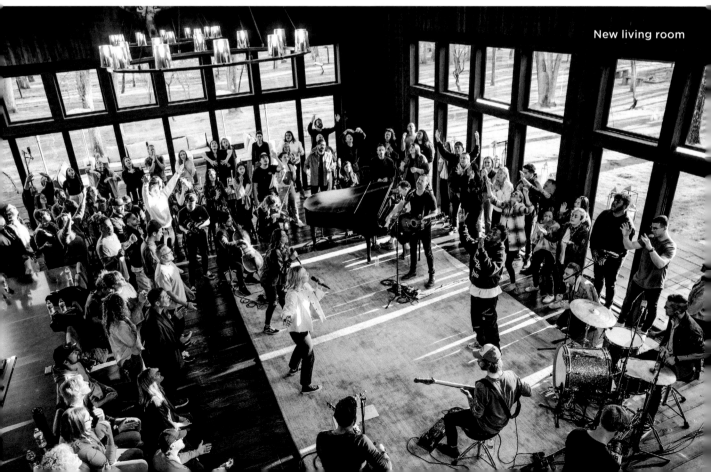

New living room

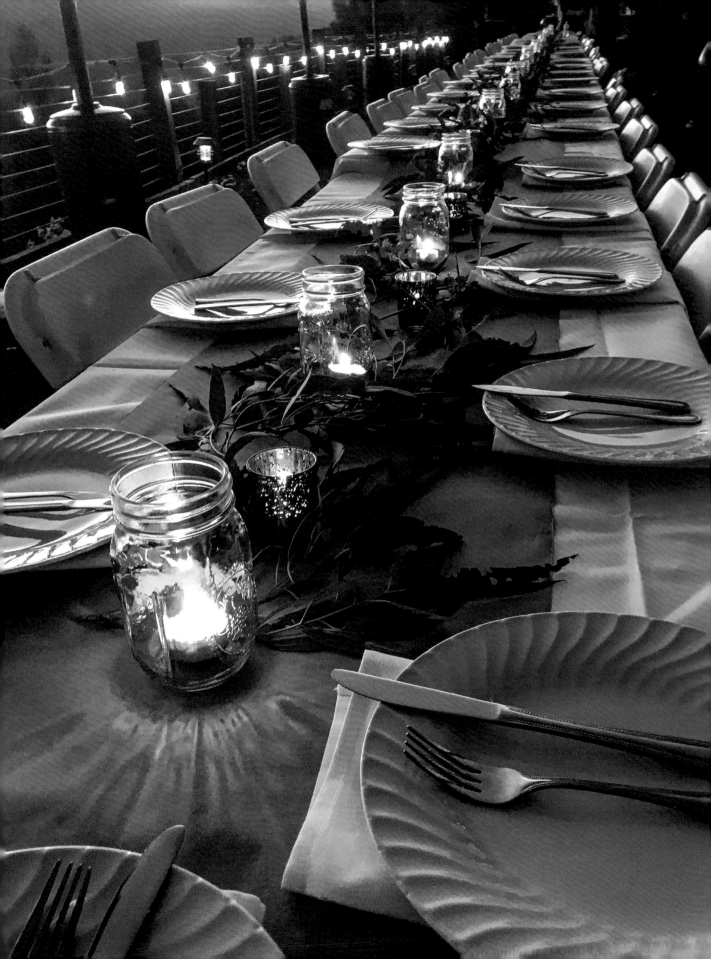

> **"Although we have structure and guidelines within our teams, the most important thing to us in navigating these relationships is encouraging each person to receive direction from the Holy Spirit."**

(We still do these monthly worship community nights to this day!)

That level of intimacy in our house changed everything; it made the team members close, like a family. We cared about each other and that was a huge part of how we were able to lead together. To encourage a way of doing life together, where a group of people put everything on the table, didn't hold things back or suffer silently, and could celebrate each other's victories. Gathering like this helped people avoid isolation and weirdness. Talking about things openly as a team helped to build trust and clear the air in tough situations.

We've made those worship community nights a priority and although we love freedom, we also love structure, so there are guidelines. In order to be on the team you are asked to commit to two practical things in addition to your spiritual life: church every Sunday (unless you are traveling), and attending team night once a month. As a record label, Bethel Music has a commitment to local church and we have fought hard to maintain healthy boundaries. It's one of the reasons we started Bethel Music.

We've seen a lot of unhealthy people in the Christian music industry; musicians living their lives on the road, many times not connected to churches or leadership. And it's not always from a bad heart, honestly, because to make a living as a musician is difficult, but we knew that God must have a better way. A way where musicians could have a healthy schedule so that they could be connected to their families and local churches. Many times as a label we would say no to opportunities because they would "break the bank" of marriages, families, or local church connection. There were difficult conversations with our team

members who wanted to be on the road more than we felt was prudent, but, ultimately, the balance of healthy families and healthy connections was what we fought for and what prevailed.

Although we have structure and guidelines within our teams, the most important thing to us in navigating these relationships is encouraging each person to receive direction from the Holy Spirit and also to talk openly with us. Whether it's a financial, personal, or professional matter, we want our team members to share whatever is on their hearts with us. Creating this environment of freedom and open communication has led to healthier relationships and deeper connections.

Now that we have a global team, with people all over the world, we do getaway retreats, team days, and songwriting retreats to **fight for and maintain those connections**. We try to be intentional and grab dinner together while we are on the road; and we FaceTime people just to check in and stay connected to them from wherever we are. With such a large team, it's difficult to truly stay connected to everybody as much as we'd love to. Instead of letting that overwhelm us, though, we ask the Holy Spirit to put people on our hearts who need connection, and we encourage our team to reach out if they need anything . . . even if it's just to talk. We have a lot of incredible pastoral people available so that even if one of our main leadership team members can't meet, our people always have someone they can talk to. Caring for people is what matters to me more than most things. Even today, since we often get asked how Bethel Music maintains its "community" and connectedness, we point to the practical behaviors and the intentionality behind them.

You might not be leading a team, but you're

connected to a team of some sort (your family, roommates, a work or church team, etc.). Maybe you're a youth pastor wanting more connection with the teenagers you lead. If you want healthy teams and members who want to stay on your teams over the long haul, apply the same concepts: provide a space to hang out and great food, invite people over, have honest (sometimes difficult) conversations, encourage, pray together, and worship . . . community.

Worshipping with the goal of God fixing things or helping us is never our aim. However, when we magnify God and worship Him, that happens. Many times as a team we have gone through difficult periods, and just gathering together to worship and focus on God has helped unify us and given us wisdom on what to do simultaneously. It's this kind of environment, community gathered in the presence of God, that brings emotional, spiritual, and physical healing.

Verses to meditate on:

When God's people are in need, be ready to help them. Always be eager to practice hospitality.

Romans 12:13 NLT

Keep on loving each other as brothers and sisters. Don't forget to show hospitality to strangers, for some who have done this have entertained angels without realizing it!

Hebrews 13:1–2 NLT

And do not forget to do good and to share with others, for with such sacrifices God is pleased.

Hebrews 13:16

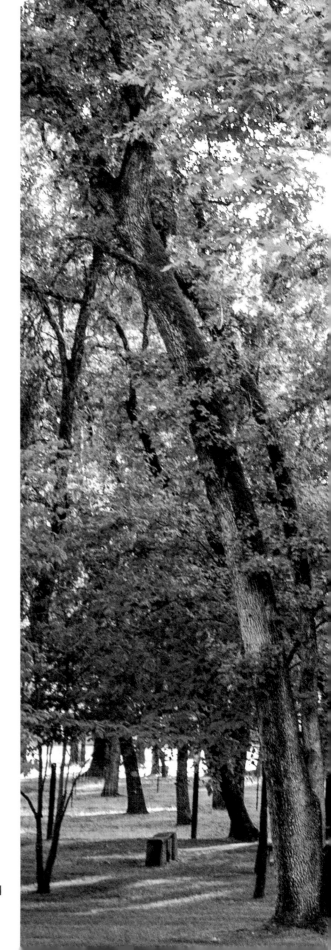

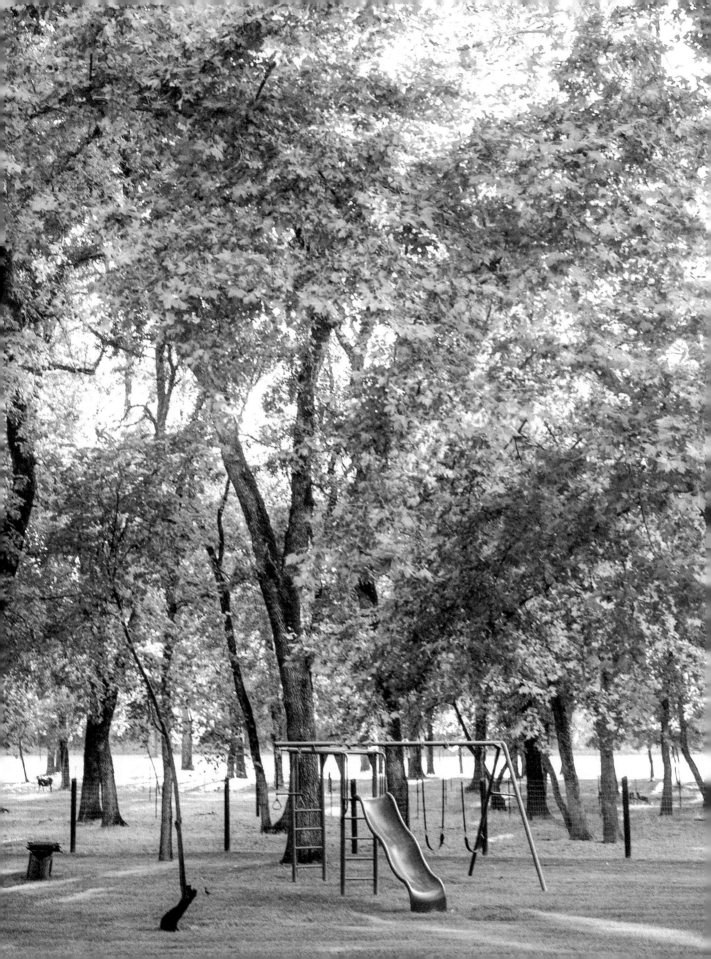

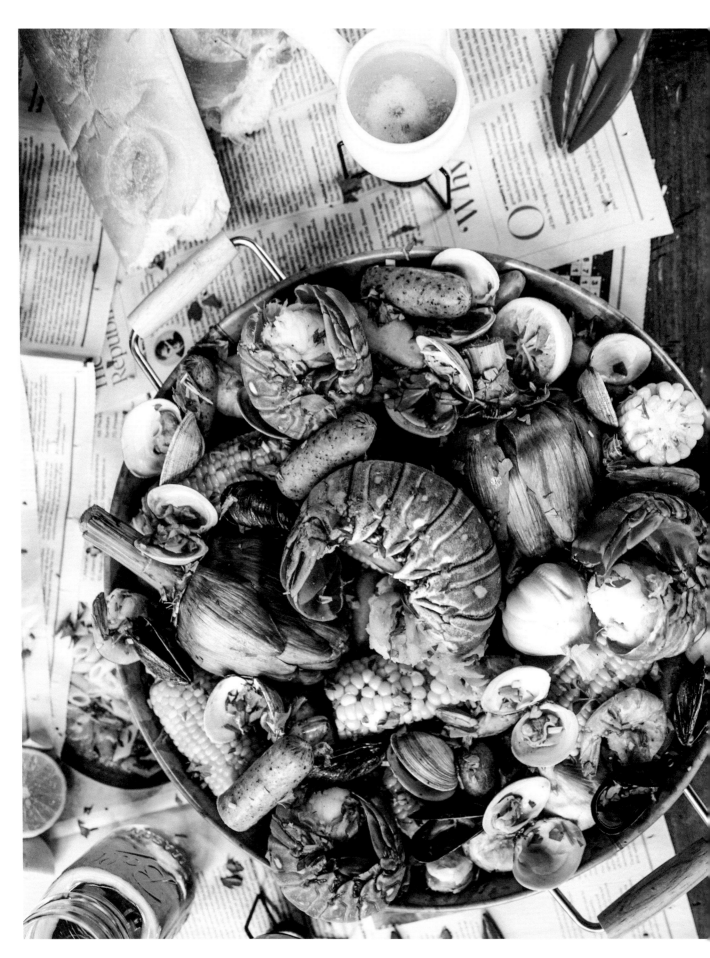

Seafood Boil

6 lemons

½ cup Old Bay seasoning, plus more for garnish

15 garlic cloves, peeled and smashed

1 onion, peeled and cut into 4 pieces

4 raw artichokes, with 1 inch of the tops cut off

1 pound small potatoes

3 lobster tails

1 pound clams, scrubbed

4 ears corn on the cob, shucked and cut in half

1 pound mussels, scrubbed

1 pound shrimp, deveined (tails on)

1 pound sausage (or chicken), cooked and cut into 4-inch pieces

4 tablespoons chopped parsley

Sourdough baguette

4 sticks of butter, melted (for dipping)

Cover your table with newspaper. Cut 4 of the lemons in half. Slice the remaining 2 lemons into wedges and place on the newspaper.

Fill a large pot with 16 cups of water. Squeeze the 4 cut lemons into the water and then add the squeezed-out lemon rinds to the pot. Next add the Old Bay seasoning, garlic, and onion. Bring to a boil.

Add the artichokes and potatoes to the pot and cook for about 10 minutes. Add the lobster tails and cook about 5 minutes. Add the clams, corn, and mussels and cook about 5 minutes. Add the shrimp and sausage (or chicken) and cook about 2 to 3 minutes. Turn off the heat.

Using tongs, take out a little bit of everything, depending on how many people you have, and put it on a serving tray. (Leave the rest in the pot to stay hot.) Sprinkle chopped parsley and Old Bay seasoning over the top. Serve immediately with sourdough baguette and melted butter . . . lots of melted butter!

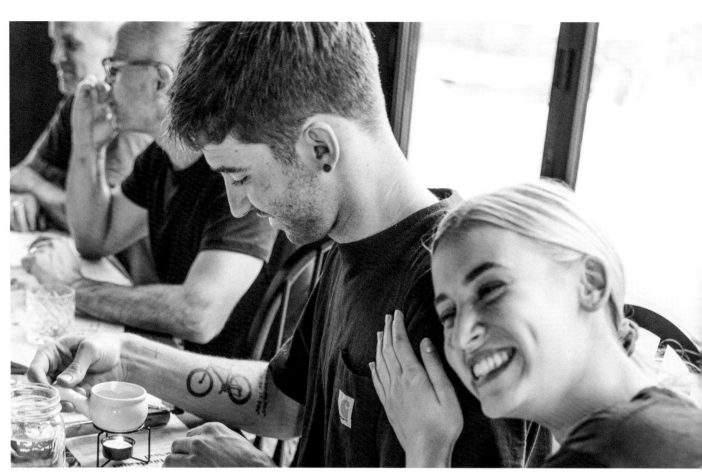

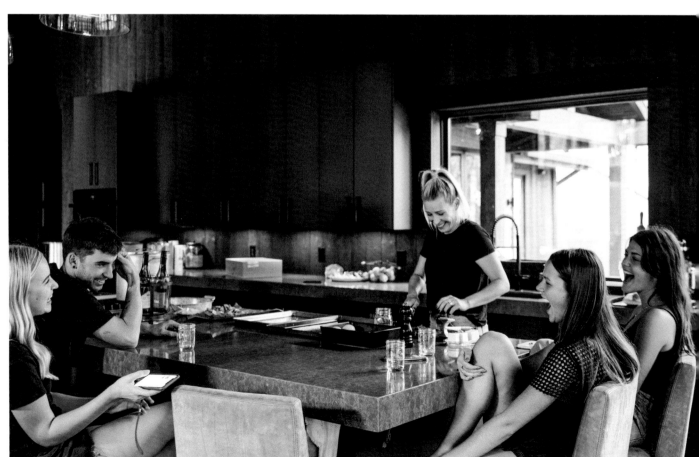

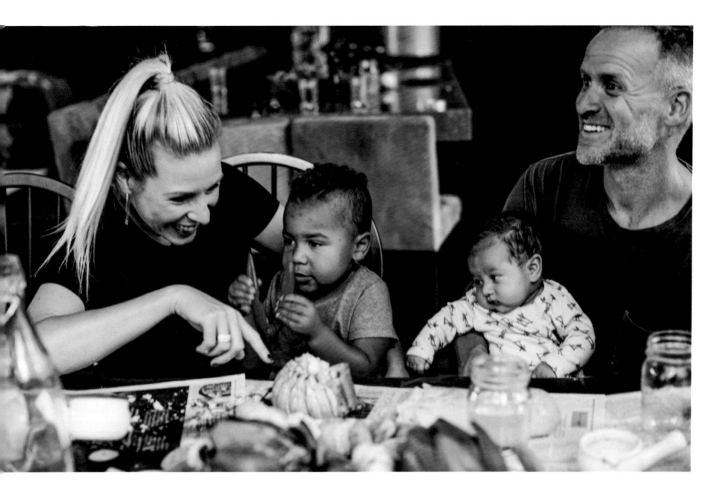

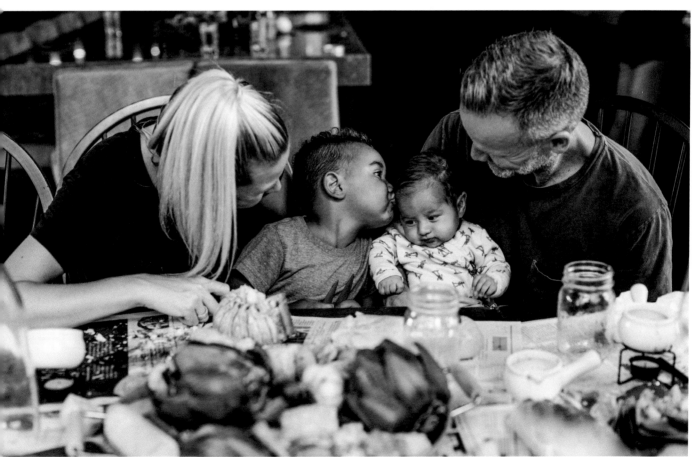

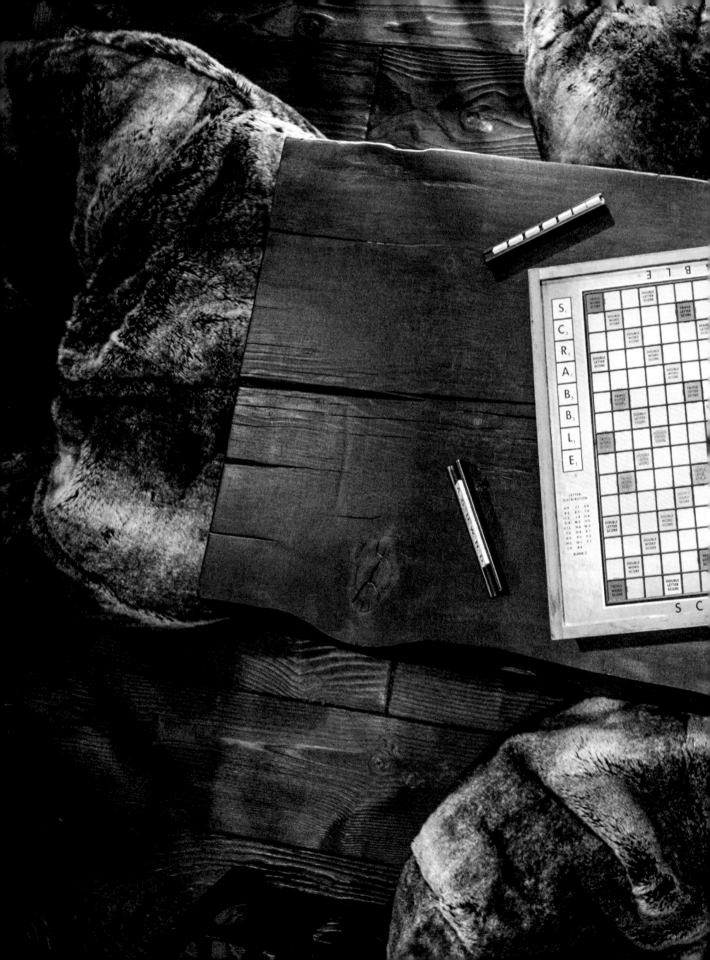

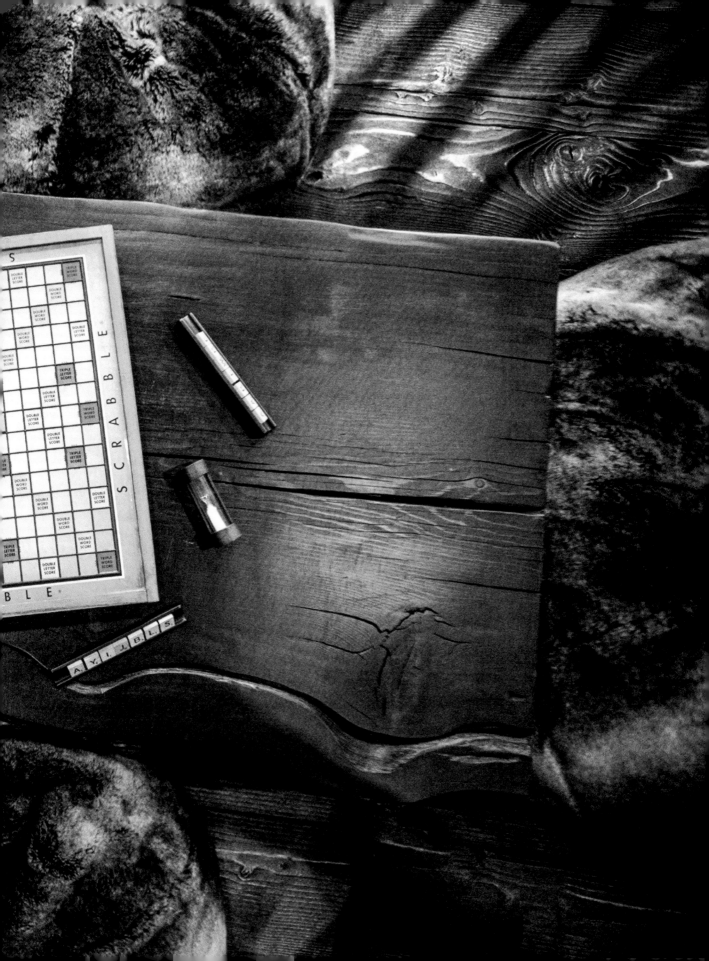

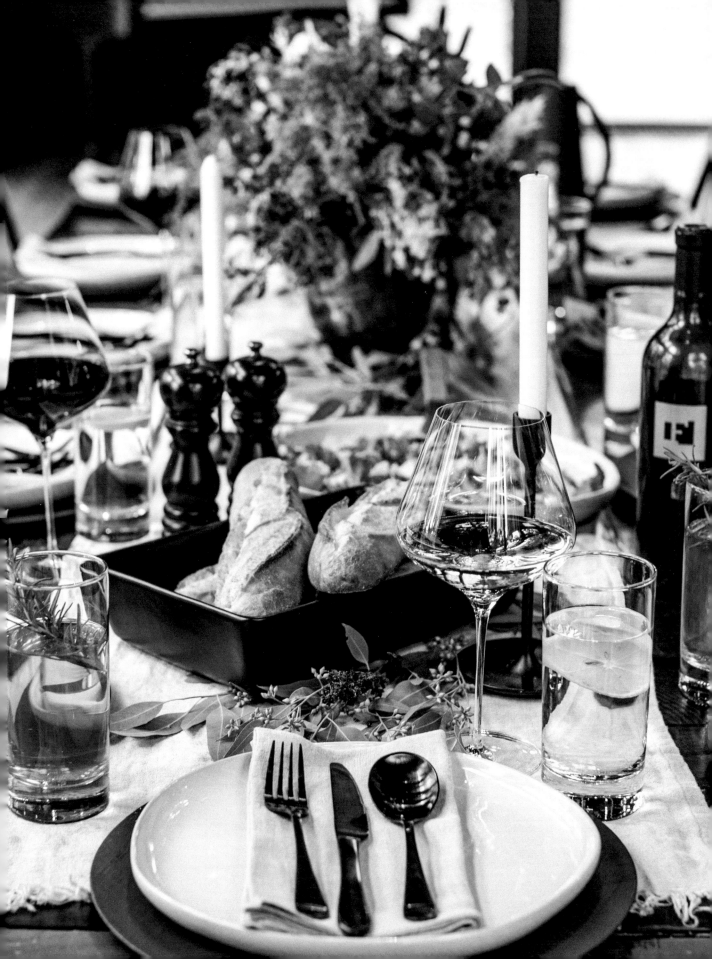

HOSTING

Whether you are new to hosting or experienced, I hope this next part of the book inspires you with creative ways that also offer money-saving options to feed and host large groups.

But no matter who you are, if you bring people together and "love from the center of who you are" (Rom. 12:9 MSG), you're off to a great start. Open your heart and home—and simply love people.

Do you need a huge home? Nope. We've hosted in all seasons of our lives and in all sizes and shapes of houses. Even in the midst of major construction, while the hammering was in the background of the party . . . we still hosted. (Not my favorite, but you make it work.) Do you need lots of money? Nope. Have everyone bring food to share. Do you need tons of friends? Not at all. Throwing parties or simple gatherings is one of the best ways to *make* friends. Do you need to be an extroverted host? Nope. Just be who you are, invite people into your home, and love them.

I want to share some basic tips and tricks with you to help make hosting easier and more fun for you, and then I want to walk you through some of my favorite events to host and hopefully inspire you to take some of my ideas and find your own traditions!

THREE LIFESAVING HOSTING TIPS

Tip 1: Stay stocked. If you're going to be gathering people regularly (which I encourage you to do . . . even if you keep it small!), it's helpful to have a specific cabinet, closet, or shelf that's stocked for your hospitality needs. That way, inviting people over last-minute won't stress you out. Always have on hand: paper plates, bowls, and cups; disposable silverware; and paper napkins. I know disposable isn't ideal, but let's be honest, dreading the cleanup is real.

pro TIP If your life feels too full for hosting, just keep it *really* simple—group text your invite, order food or have everyone bring something to share, put out your disposable dinnerware, and throw on some background music (like some quality instrumental jazz!). Ask a friend or two to help you set up and a friend or two to clean up. Even if they're just staying thirty extra minutes, you'll be thankful. You don't have to do it all. **Ask for help!**

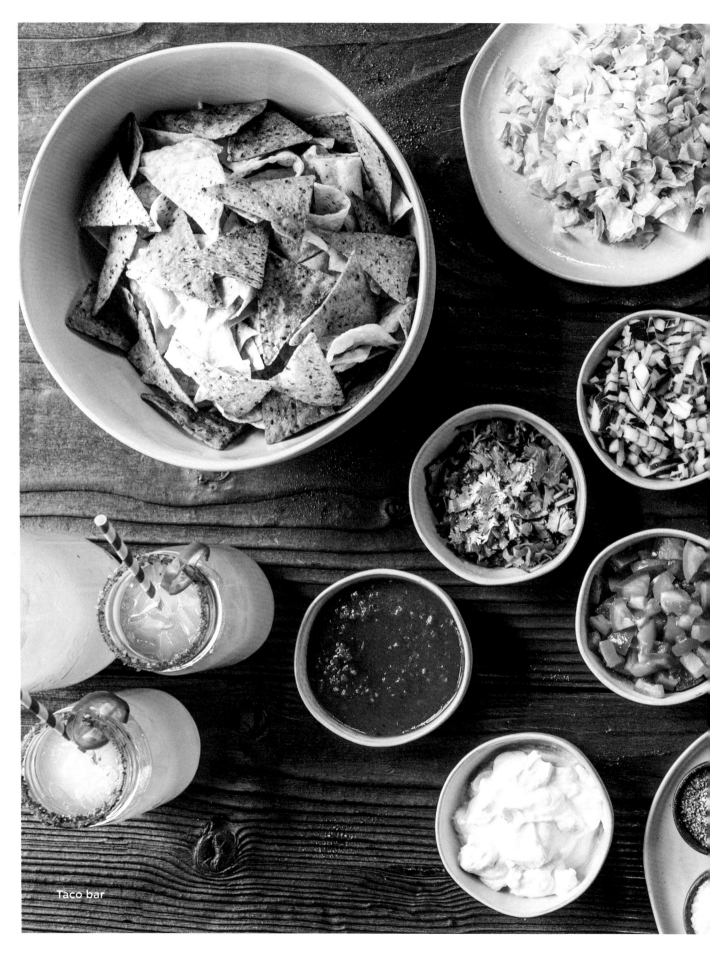

Taco bar

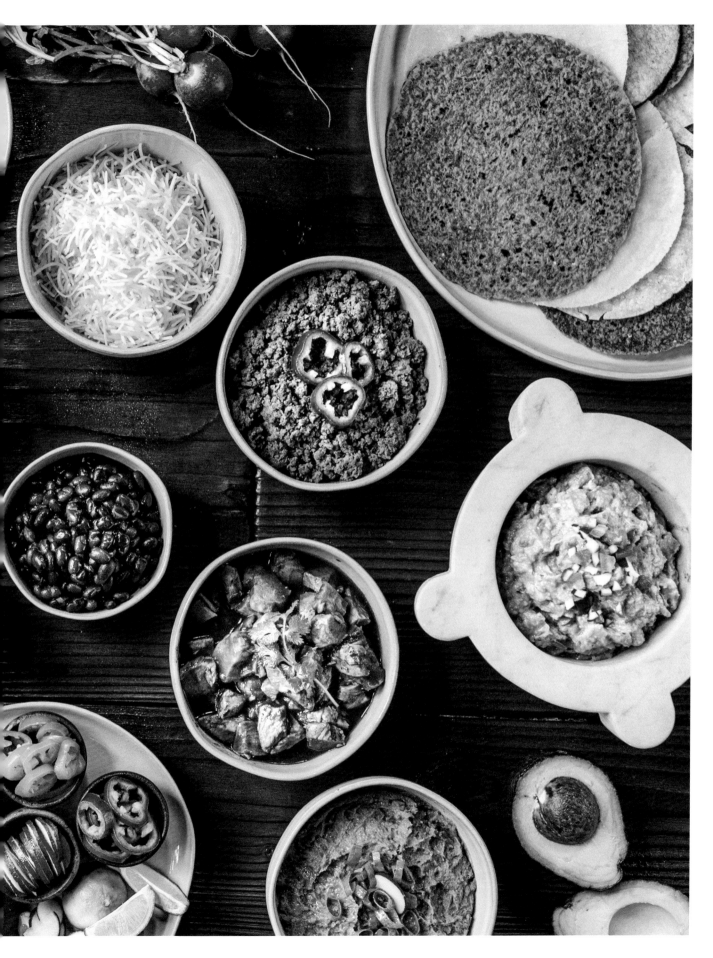

Tip 2: Make cleanup simple. Ease of cleaning up can make the difference of *actually* having people over or not. This go-to stockpile of disposable plates, bowls, cups, silverware, and napkins helps take the pressure off each time you host, because you know where everything is, and you can just pull it off the shelf when you're ready. Staying organized makes it easy to tell what you're out of and need to replace. (And, like most things, if you want to take it a step further with order, put these supplies in labeled containers.)

Tip 3: Food bars! One of my favorite things to do for a party is a food bar—it's a game changer when hosting. You take a food theme—let's say, tacos—and create a table spread that has all the staples, multiple meat and tortilla options, and as many toppings (jalapeños, onions, refried beans, black beans, cilantro, avocado, olives, sour cream, hot sauce, radishes, limes, pepitas, cotija, Monterey Jack, cheddar, and nacho cheese) as you can think of. Your guests get to customize their meal to their personal preference, which makes everyone happy. They can go simple or gourmet, and you don't have to plan meal alternatives for any picky eaters. Food bars let your guests eat the way *they* want and at the end of this chapter, I'm sharing some of my favorites!

THE SINGLES MIXER

In traveling for twenty years while practicing ministry, we've met so many incredible, Spirit-filled people who, for one reason or another, aren't married. Many of them are single because they simply haven't found the right person yet. The point is, there are many incredible single Christians all over the world! And many of them live in the same city and don't even know one another. Such a diverse group too: some are young, some are older, some are famous. Some of these people have told me how they often questioned if something was wrong with them (not a thing), and how lonely they often

feel. But putting the description "Christian" into an online dating site can mean SO many things (or . . . nothing!). Many of my friends were wanting to date and meet new people, they just needed a chance to connect. So, I had an idea: Why not invite all of my amazing single friends from all over the world to our house for a party!? I made a digital invite that read something like this:

> *Here's the deal. I have so many incredible, Spirit-filled, single friends (just like you) around the world who haven't met the right person yet. So, I'm throwing a party and you're invited. Come meet other amazing single people (ages 18–75 and all approved by me or someone I'm close friends with) at our house for a laid-back, fun evening. Attire is dressy-casual, and please bring $25 for food & drinks. You'll meet many amazing people and maybe you'll meet someone special! RSVP soon so I can get a head count for food. Love you!*

The response was amazing—more than one hundred people RSVP'd within minutes, and then more! (The guys were a little slower to respond, but not slow to show up!) People all over started to hear about it and asked if they could come, but in order to attend the mixer, they had to be personally recommended by me or someone I knew and trusted.

As we got closer to the date, I enlisted a few married friends to help me on the day of the event with parking, running a registration table, serving food, and cleaning up. (These married friends still love getting involved, and once they hear I'm throwing a singles party, they often offer to help before I even have to ask. It's fun people-watching.)

On the morning of the first event, I made enough chili to feed an army. One chili with meat and one without for the vegetarians. I did a "chili bar" (yay, food bars) with bowls of corn chips, tortilla chips, and toppings (just like in the taco bar). To get the registration table ready, I printed out three

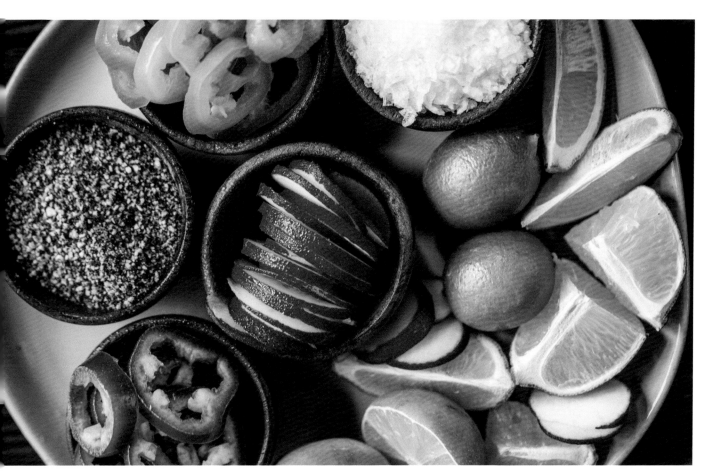

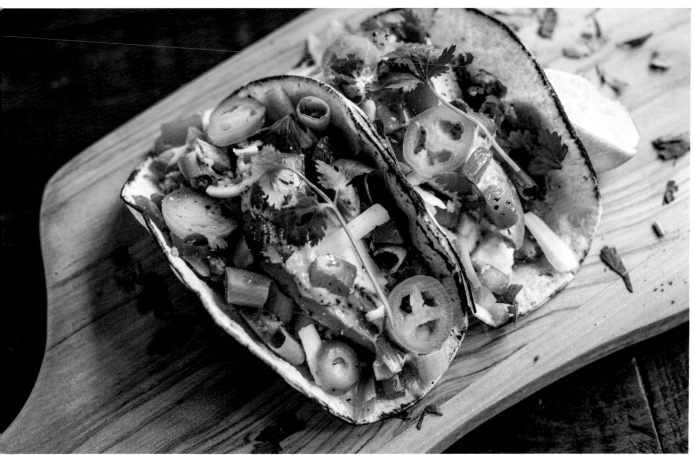

If there are great singles in your community you want to introduce to one another, a singles mixer is a great alternative to awkward blind dates. Here are my ten steps for throwing a great singles mixer:

1| Create an online invite (I use Evite). Take a screenshot of it, send it to all your trusted friends, and ask them to text the invite to any amazing, healthy, Spirit-filled Christian single people they know.

2| Plan your food and drinks (ideas at the end of this chapter).

3| Buy some paper wristbands and adhesive name tags.

4| Create a playlist.

5| Collect tables (I use picnic tables and cocktail tables) and chairs and supplies: disposable plates, cups, napkins, and silverware; candles.

6| Ask a few married friends to help with parking, registration, cooking, food setup, and cleanup.

7| While people are registering, allow about thirty minutes for a simple "Hey, tell me about you!" quick conversation time.

8| Rally everyone together with a quick pep talk: "You're all amazing! This is a safe space! Ask someone out after this!"

9| Break everyone into some sort of age grouping, then further into smaller groups of six or seven. Each small group will have its own conversation where everyone goes around and shares their name, where they live and work, and one additional thing about themselves. You can have each person hold a minute timer ("when it's done, you're done," and pass it on) so that no one hogs the conversation. After each person has shared, the guys move to the next group, but the ladies stay. Do this until everyone has mixed.

10| Encourage the singles to eat together, mingle, and . . . ask people out!

It's as simple as that! Hosting a singles mixer is a beautiful way of loving and encouraging the singles community.

copies of the list of people registered and put them on the table with marker pens, name tags, and wristbands for check-in. (I knew people would try to sneak in . . . and they did. Gotcha!) I put out disposable cups, labeled and filled large dispensers with ice water and hot apple cider, and turned on a great playlist (curated by my daughter) through the outdoor speakers. I had a few corn hole games set up, and cards and other games on picnic tables throughout the yard. Last, I had outdoor lights and real candles in lanterns all over the place for the romance vibes.

Once people showed up, they got checked in to make sure their name was on the list, and then they got a wristband and a name tag to fill out. We had them put their name and Instagram handle on their tag so people could easily find them afterward to connect. Then we directed them to get a drink, encouraged them to talk to someone they'd like to get to know and offered a simple conversation starter: "So, tell me about you!"

Thirty minutes later, once everyone was checked in, I gathered them for a "pep talk": "Listen, you're all amazing and this is a safe place. Get to know each other. Make friends *and* look for a spouse. And ask people out after this!"

I talked through the mixer instructions. I told them they would be divided into age groups (18–35 and 36+) for the first part of the mixer. Then they would gather in smaller groups of 7 (4 girls, 3 guys . . . the women outnumbered the men a little). I told them to go around in the small groups and each tell their name, where they lived and worked, and one additional thing about themselves. Every five minutes a bell went off, and the guys moved down to the next group and the girls stayed in place, and so on, until they'd all mixed. After that (about an hour) we served dinner . . . chili bar! I encouraged them to talk to the people they were attracted to during the first part of the mixer and say something like, "I'd love to get to know you better." (Honestly, giving people a scripted line to say seems to work

really well and breaks the ice. Even if it's a repeated thing throughout the mixer . . . it actually makes the atmosphere lighthearted and fun.) After dinner, the mixer was organic; I told people to be courageous and ask anyone they were attracted to out on a dessert date or coffee date the next day to get to know them more.

It was such a great night! All those amazing people walking into the backyard, looking great, nervous, and excited (or as my daughter Téa calls it, "nervocited"; ha!). There was such a present sense of hope. Many of those attending had been fighting loneliness and depression, but that night they laughed and shared stories with other amazing people just like them in *a place where they felt comfortable.* (I've thrown the singles mixer party many times now, and I find ways to make it better each year!)

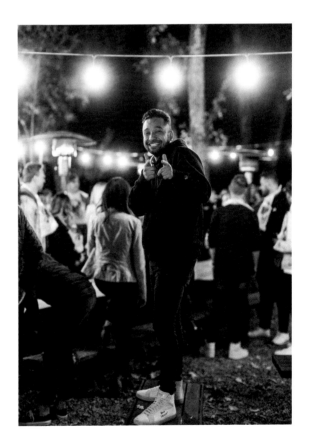

Chili

1 tablespoon olive oil

1 medium onion, diced

1 pound lean ground beef

2½ tablespoons chili powder

2 tablespoons ground cumin

2 tablespoons tomato paste

1 tablespoon garlic powder

1½ teaspoons salt

½ teaspoon ground black pepper

¼ teaspoon ground cayenne pepper

1 (15-ounce) can San Marzano diced tomatoes, blended

1 (16-ounce) can red kidney beans, drained and rinsed

1 (16-ounce) can pinto beans

1½ cups beef broth

1 (8-ounce) can tomato sauce

Baked potatoes (for serving)

Another annual party we host is our **Super Bowl party**—the perfect time for a food bar. It's all about the salty snacks, dips, and root beer floats. (And halftime is a great opportunity to get seconds, since the halftime show is usually raunchy.) We invite a few families and friends over every year after church and everyone brings something to share. Ice-cold drinks and tons of yummy food while we watch the game and the kids play outside—it's the best. If the weather is nice, I keep the food covered on a table in a shaded area of the lawn so the chickens, and not me, can clean up around the table.

Heat the oil in a large Dutch oven or pot over medium-high heat. Add the diced onion and cook 4 to 5 minutes. Add the ground beef and stir, breaking it into very small pieces; cook for about 5 minutes. Add the chili powder, cumin, tomato paste, garlic powder, salt, pepper, and cayenne. Stir well. Add the tomatoes, beans, beef broth, and tomato sauce. Stir well. Turn heat to low and simmer 25 to 30 minutes.

Serve chili with tons of topping options like:

- shredded cheese (cheddar or Mexican blend)
- sliced green onions
- chopped cilantro
- diced avocado
- tamed jalapeños
- corn chips
- tortilla chips

Serve over a baked potato.

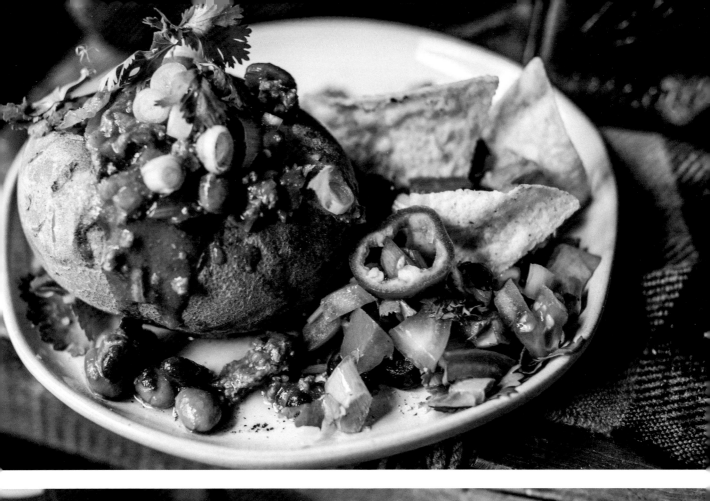
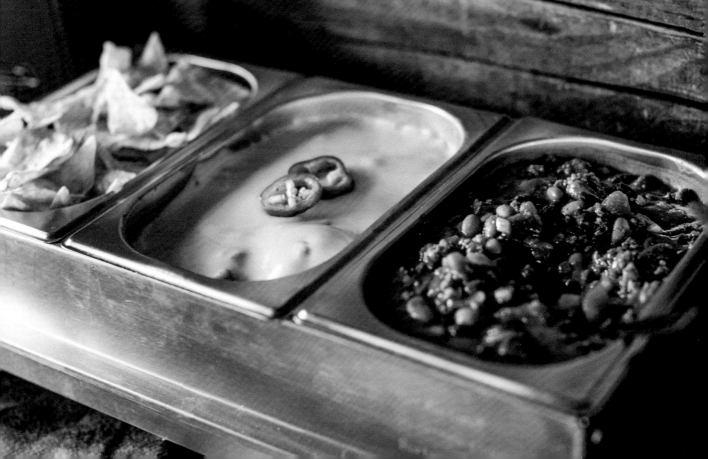

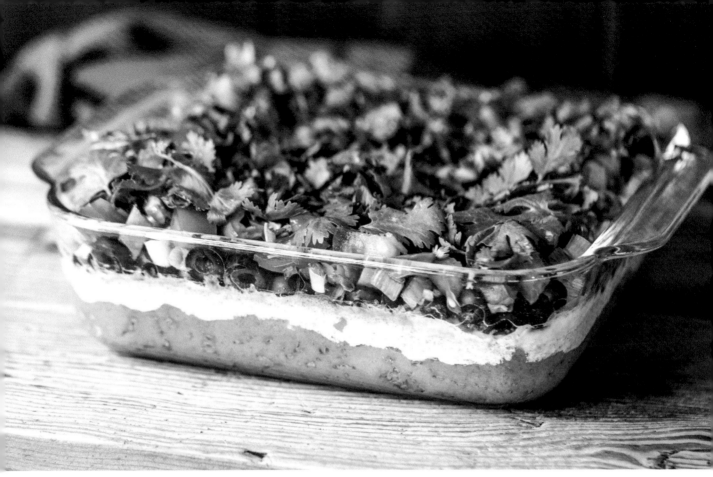

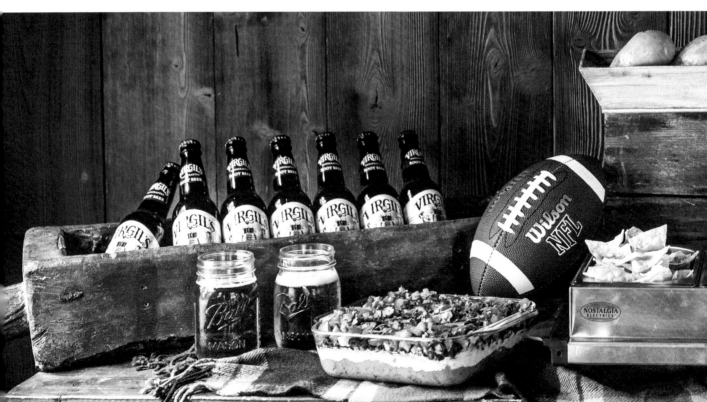

Taco Dip

1 (16-ounce) can refried beans

8 ounces cream cheese, softened

1 cup sour cream

2 tablespoons taco seasoning mix

2 garlic cloves, peeled and minced

½ cup shredded cheddar cheese

½ cup sliced black olives

1 medium tomato, chopped

3 green onions, chopped

2 tablespoons chopped cilantro

Tortilla chips and/or corn chips

Preheat the oven to 350°F. Spread the beans over the bottom of an 8 x 8-inch baking pan. Combine the cream cheese, sour cream, taco seasoning, and garlic in a medium bowl. Spread the cream cheese mixture over the beans. Bake for 15 to 18 minutes, or until hot. Remove the pan from the oven and top with cheddar cheese. Return the pan to the oven and bake an additional 2 to 3 minutes, or until the cheese has melted.

Sprinkle the olives, tomato, green onions, and cilantro over the dip. Serve with tortilla chips and/or corn chips.

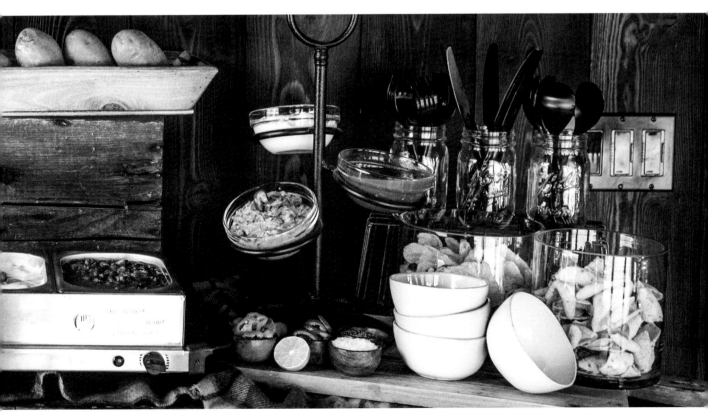

Hosting

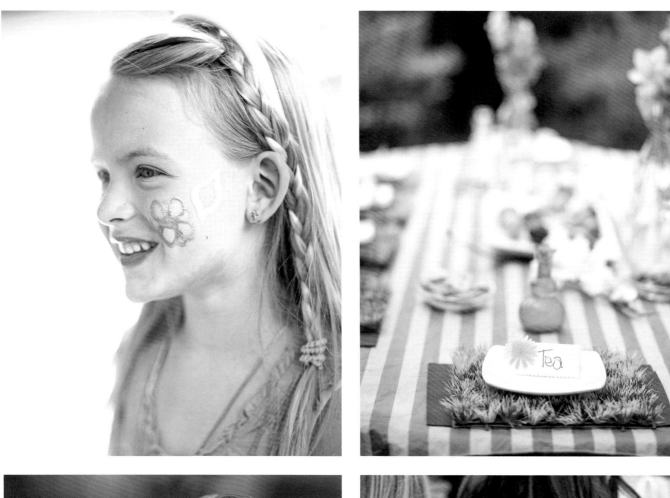

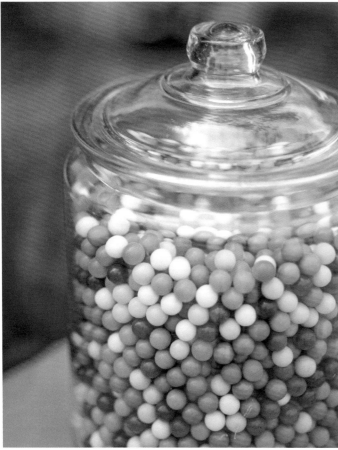

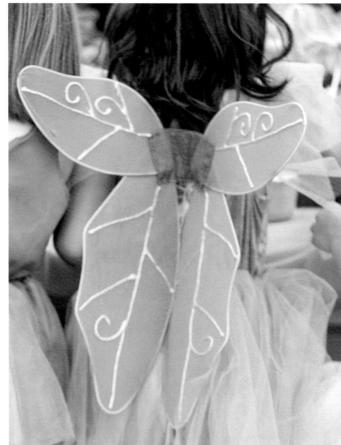

KIDS' BIRTHDAY PARTIES

I go over the top with birthday parties for my kids. I love celebrating them and making the day as "all about them" as possible. (You only turn that age once, right?) This doesn't mean we spend a lot of money, though! I get really resourceful and creative. The kids feel extra love through the intentionality of the party.

About a month before the birthday of one of our kids, I ask them to tell me about their dream party: what theme, snacks, and games they'd like. Having five kids, we've done a *million* themes: princesses, superheroes, forest fairies, Blue's Clues, Strawberry Shortcake, Hannah Montana, LEGO, Super Mario, horses, dinosaurs, and more!

Once I know their theme, I start looking online for inspiration (thank you, Pinterest). I go extravagant but thrifty—often borrowing things from friends or renting items we don't have instead of buying. Some years we've had the parties at a local park (when we didn't have the backyard space), or at a party specialty store, which is also a great idea because it keeps the mess out of your house/yard, but since we have a pool and a big yard now, we usually host everything at our home.

I let the kids invite all their friends . . . and sometimes their whole school class comes! It's wild, but why not, right? We create an online invite together that reveals the theme of the party and details (with a note that says, "You can drop your child off at 3 and pick them up at 5," as a hint that we don't need parents to stay because that would mean thirty to sixty more people). I print enough invites for the whole class so the kids can pass them out. I text the invite to our family as well.

Then I create a gift registry. (I've talked about this in the "Room by Room" chapter, but basically I do a registry so people have an idea of what the birthday boy or girl would love and it has really been helpful! I love knowing what someone wants so I can buy it for them. Takes the guesswork out.) For my older kids, instead of registering, they like to create a "Present Ideas" board on Pinterest of what they want, including sizes and colors. I use it to shop for them and then share the rest with our family members who want ideas! Works great, they're still surprised, and you have *way* fewer returns. Giving gifts is definitely a love language for many people in our huge family, and Christmas is crazy with forty-plus people to buy for in the company and family, so . . . this really helps!

Even though we eat healthy, birthday parties are a time for cheating! We have good food options, too, but I make it a point to let the kids have whatever unhealthy stuff they want. Doughnuts, Cheetos, candy, ice cream . . . we go for it.

The day of the party, I decorate the outdoor area and tables in the party theme and fill a huge container with lemonade. When all the guests arrive, we just keep things simple: play, swim if it's warm enough, eat snacks, sing happy birthday, eat dessert, open presents! We have a swing set, a trampoline, and a bunch of sporting equipment, and we let the kids run wild. I'm not a huge fan of organized games, so I love to let the kids run free while I sit back and enjoy a glass of lemonade after the hard work of planning the party. It's usually a million kids running around having the time of their lives in our backyard and Brian and I refilling snacks and drinking lemonade while hanging out with our family. It's the best.

---

pro TIP

Regifting! If we get something we don't need (be honest), we're big on regifting. Some people have a hard time with regifting, but if you or your child doesn't love the gift . . . don't keep it. (And the same goes for adults' gifts.) Keep what you love and give away what you don't—bless someone else. **Let. It. Go.**

BARBECUES AND POOL PARTIES

These are my favorite. Outdoor, casual, chill gatherings. Now that we have a pool, we love to share it . . . and we do almost every day of the summer. (We didn't have one the first fifteen years of our marriage and the temperature where we live is frequently over 115 degrees . . . it's incredible to have one now!) But pool or not, a casual backyard hangout is a fun way to bring people together— especially if there's some fun activity to do, like badminton, making s'mores, corn hole, swimming, or volleyball. And let's be honest, for hanging out with other families with kids, backyard parties save your house from being destroyed by the kids while the parents hang out.

I'm obsessed with fresh lemonade, so our backyard parties almost always have a huge container of it: fresh lemon juice, agave nectar, water, and ice. I also love to refrigerate cubed watermelon and serve it with fresh squeezed lime juice and a little sea salt on it. I feed the watermelon rinds to our chickens and the wild deer. They love them. Some of our favorite poolside foods are: carrots and hummus, chips and salsa, and lentils and bruschetta (recipe on page 195). Just keep the food covered and on ice. Nobody wants warm hummus or bugs in their food. (I use metal mesh covers.) And when we host around lunch or dinner, a go-to is our "burger bar" with my grandma Jane's potato salad recipe! I love letting people create their own burgers (beef, turkey, or vegetarian), with tons of topping options like tomatoes, lettuce, pickles, onions, jalapeños, mushrooms, cheese, bacon, mayo, ketchup, and mustard.

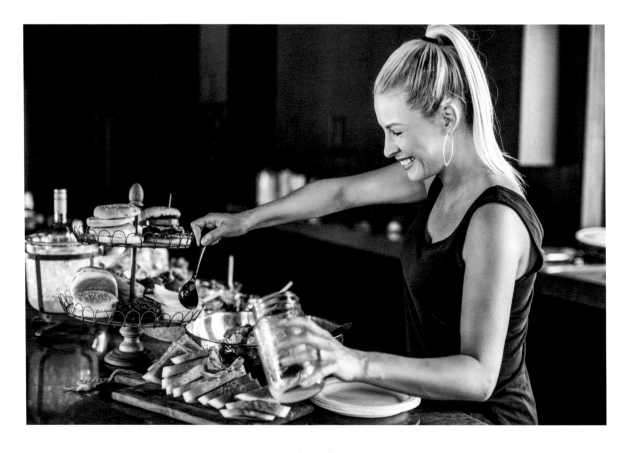

Grandma Jane's Potato Salad

25 baby creamer potatoes

1 cup chopped dill pickles

10 eggs, hard-boiled and chopped

½ cup mayonnaise

⅓ cup Dijon mustard

1 teaspoon black pepper

1½ teaspoons salt

4 pieces bacon, cooked and chopped

2 green onions, chopped

Put the potatoes in a large stockpot, cover them with cold water and add a generous amount of salt. Boil the potatoes until they're tender, drain them, and put them in a large bowl. (Cut them in half or leave them whole.) Add pickles, eggs, mayonnaise, mustard, black pepper, salt, bacon, and green onions. Mix until combined. Top with additional bacon, green onions, salt, and cracked black pepper.

Lentils with Bruschetta and Feta

2 cups lentils, cooked

½ teaspoon salt

½ teaspoon black pepper

10 ounces bruschetta sauce

6 ounces feta cheese

Pita chips

Mix the cooked lentils with salt and pepper. Place the lentils in the bottom of a glass dish. Layer the bruschetta on top and then the crumbled feta. Serve with pita chips.

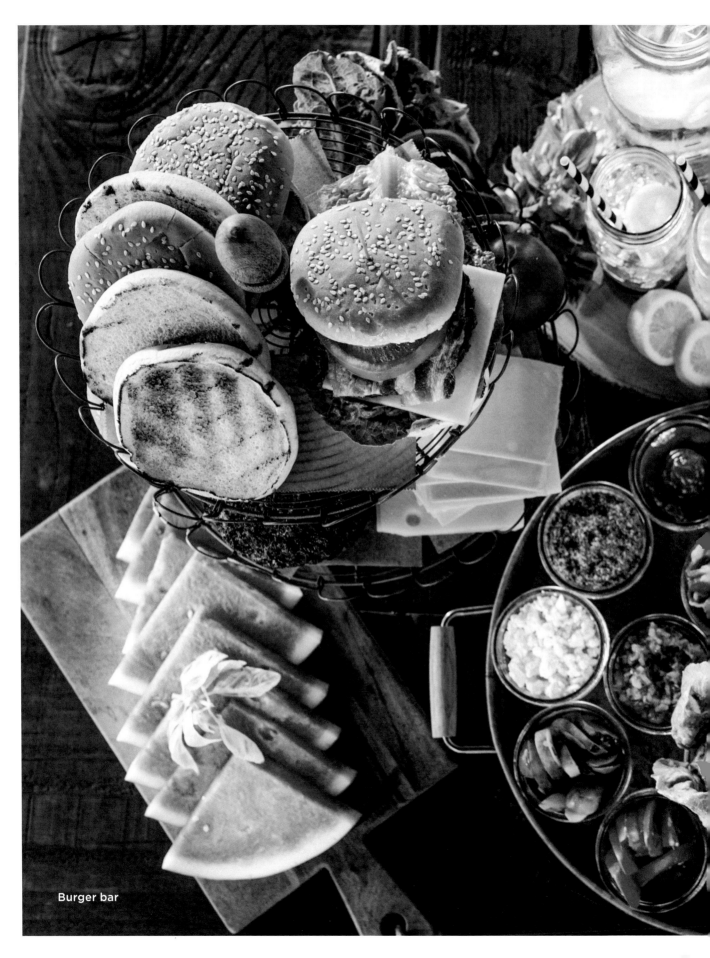
Burger bar

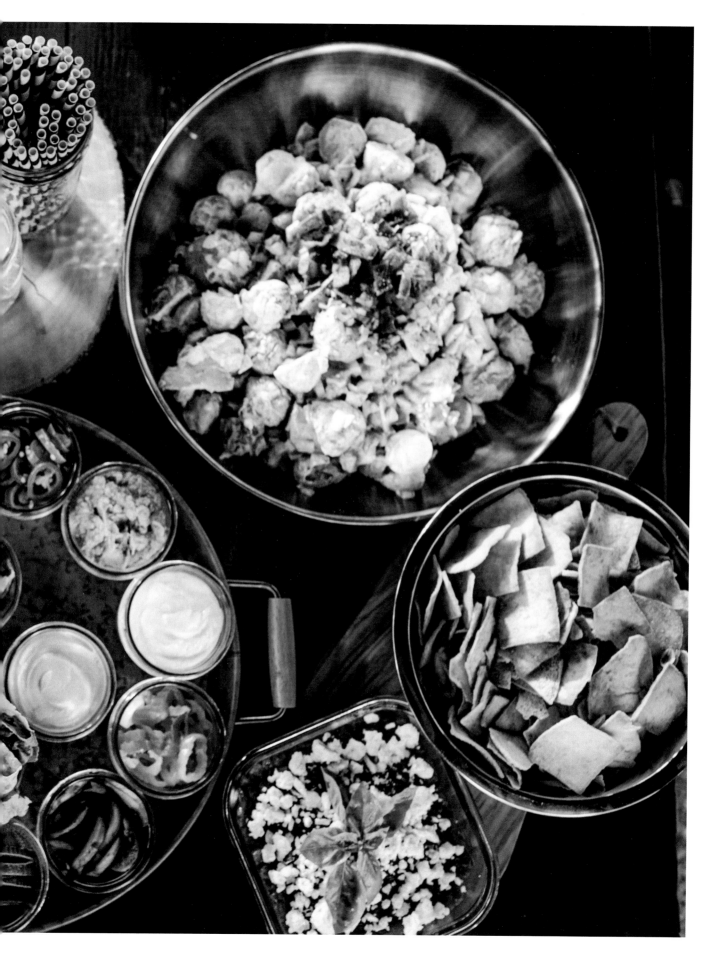

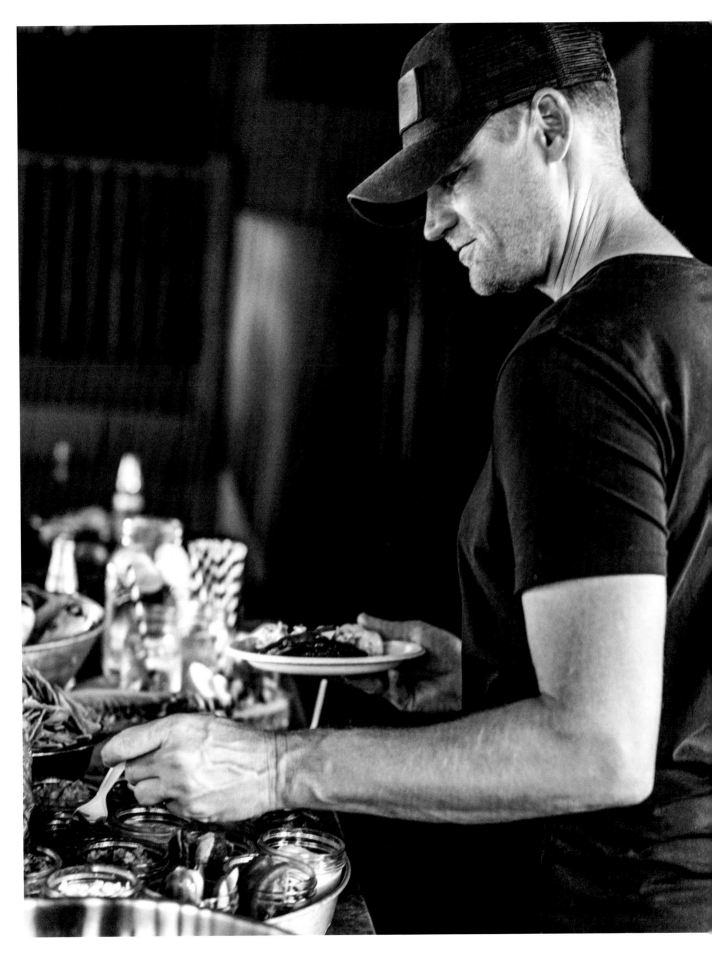

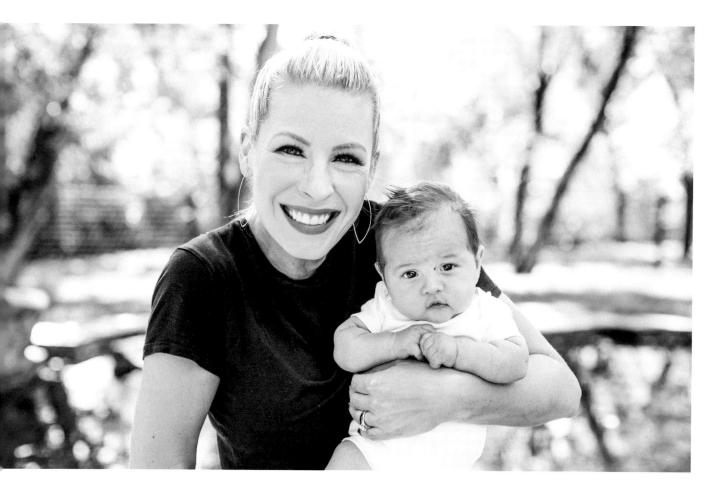
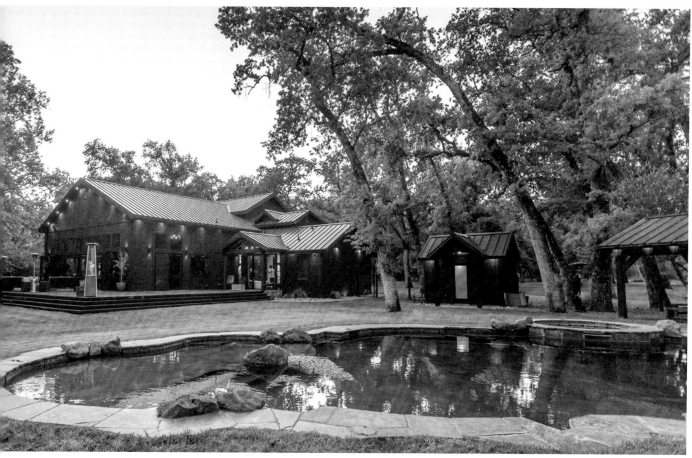

SEASONAL PARTIES

A change of seasons is a great reason to host a gathering—and maybe even make it a tradition! One I love is my **fall girlfriends' brunch**. Every year when the kids go back to school, I invite my girlfriends over to celebrate that it's fall and we made it through the summer with us and our kids still alive. Yay! I have everyone bring a brunch item to share and the more pumpkin-flavored things, the better! I brew a LOT of coffee and put out cream and agave nectar. And I make my favorite pumpkin cookies. I put vegetables in everything I can. Even dessert! These cookies are SO good (recipe opposite). I usually start it around 9:30 a.m. so everyone can get their kids to school and then swing by the store if they haven't had time to make something. And yes, Starbucks pumpkin bread is perfect. Bring it. I will eat it!

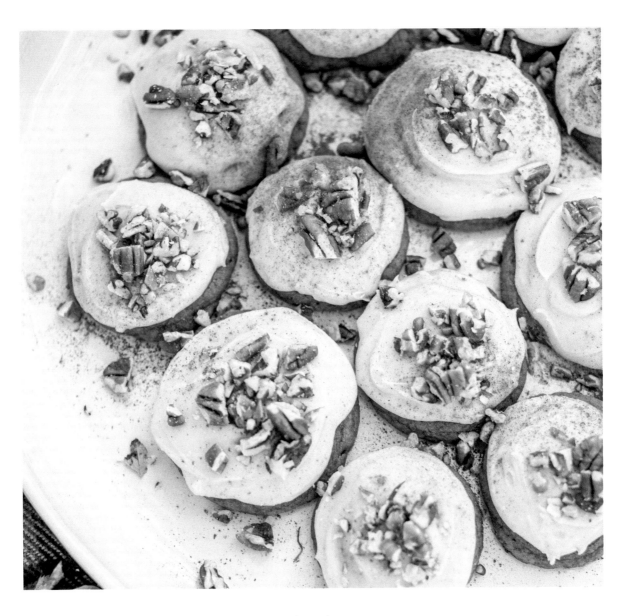

Pumpkin Cookies

2¾ cups all-purpose flour

1 teaspoon baking powder

1 teaspoon baking soda

1¼ teaspoons salt

2 teaspoons ground cinnamon

1½ teaspoons ground ginger

1 teaspoon ground nutmeg

1½ sticks salted butter, softened

2 cups light brown sugar

2 eggs

1 (15-ounce) can pumpkin

¾ cup evaporated milk

1 teaspoon bourbon vanilla extract (vanilla extract will also be fine)

ICING

4 cups powdered sugar

10 tablespoons butter, melted

5 tablespoons evaporated milk

2 teaspoons bourbon vanilla extract (or vanilla extract)

¼ teaspoon cinnamon

Preheat the oven to 375°F. Line a baking sheet with parchment paper. Mix the flour, baking powder, baking soda, salt, cinnamon, ginger, and nutmeg in a medium bowl. With a mixer, blend the butter with the brown sugar. Mix in the eggs. Then add the pumpkin, evaporated milk, and bourbon vanilla extract and mix until combined. Next add the flour mixture and mix until well combined. Use a small cookie scoop (or piping bag) and put scoops of batter on the baking sheet 1 inch apart. Bake them about 12 minutes, then let them cool for 5 minutes before transferring to a wire rack.

While the cookies are cooling, make the icing. Put the powdered sugar in a bowl. Melt 10 tablespoons of butter and pour it over the powdered sugar. Stir in the evaporated milk, bourbon vanilla extract, and cinnamon. Spread the icing on the completely cooled cookies and try not to eat ten of them at once!

pro TIP Always crack the eggs into a separate bowl before you add them to your recipe in case you have a bad egg or a stray piece of shell.

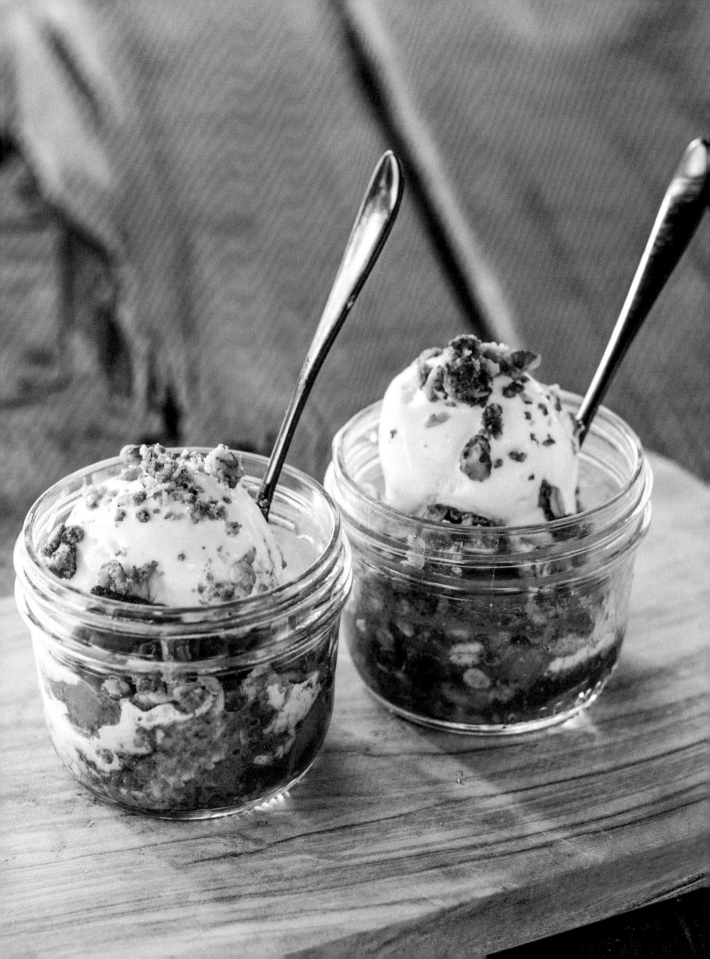

Apple Cinnamon Crumble

CRUMBLE MIXTURE

1½ cups all-purpose flour, sifted

1 cup brown sugar

1 cup rolled oats

1 cup chopped pecans

1 teaspoon salt

12 tablespoons unsalted butter, melted

Preheat the oven to 350°F and butter a 13 x 9-inch pan.

In a medium bowl, combine the flour, brown sugar, oats, pecans, and salt.

Once combined, add the melted butter and stir with a fork until all the dry ingredients are wet.

Make sure all of the big chunks are broken up.

APPLE MIXTURE

8 large Granny Smith apples

½ cup brown sugar

1 tablespoon ground cinnamon

2 tablespoons fresh lemon juice

Core each apple and chop into ½-inch pieces. Place the pieces in a large bowl and add the brown sugar, cinnamon, and lemon juice. Spread apples in an even layer in the buttered baking dish and then press the crumble mixture onto the apples until they're covered. Bake for about 60 minutes, until the crumble topping turns golden brown. (After 45 minutes, watch the bottom to make sure it's not burning.)

Serve with your favorite vanilla ice cream.

FOURTH OF JULY

Every year when I was a little girl, the Fourth of July meant four things—a huge barbecue at my uncle's house by the fishing pond, yummy trash food, playing with cousins and friends for hours, and fireworks. Those are some of my favorite memories. We don't have a pond, but the Fourth of July looks about the same for us, just around the pool instead. I send out a text that says something like this: "We'll be in the pool all day with family and friends, so come on over anytime and bring a snack to share. Just let me know if you're coming so I can get a head count for burgers." There's always tons of watermelon, country music, kids everywhere . . . and, you guessed it . . . lemonade—it's my favorite summer drink.

HALLO . . . "HARVEST PARTY!"

Although the origin and observation of Halloween is a subject for mixed opinions, it's a day that marks the end of harvest and the beginning of "the holidays" . . . the best! Growing up, we would have a church dress-up party (no scary or evil costumes allowed) on October 31, with carnival games and homemade apple cider, called the "Harvest Party." For me, a social-event lover, it was better than Christmas. We were allowed to go door-to-door collecting candy but only to the houses of people we knew. We didn't celebrate darkness, evil, or anything scary, but we redeemed the day! (Darkness wasn't going to have a day.) **We celebrated God, all things fall—pumpkin everything, caramel apples, hayrides—community, and the beginning of the holidays!** And I LOVE the holidays.

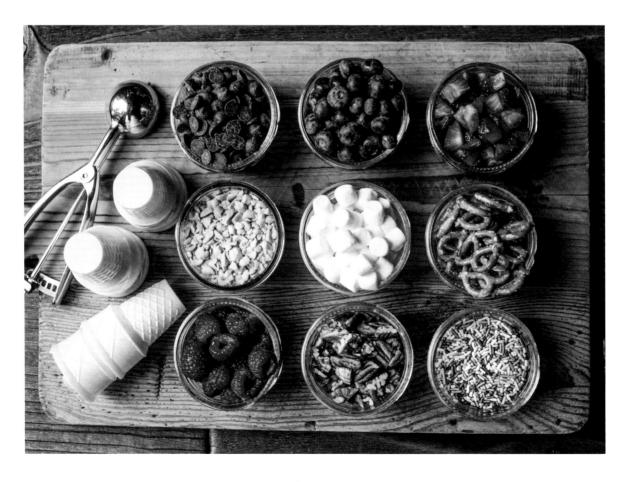

THE HOLIDAYS

When it comes to Thanksgiving and Christmas, we go all out. Since most of our family live close to us (on both sides), most years we have multiple days of celebrating Thanksgiving and Christmas with different sides of the family. Oftentimes we are asked why we don't just combine them and the answer is . . . because that would be around a hundred people. Plus, it's really fun having so much family time.

We divide up the "who's cooking what?" work among everyone and each bring something. For the Johnson holidays (there's sixty-two of us), we start in the morning with Grandma Johnson's (Amma) divine cinnamon rolls. They are truly life-changing.

For lunch, we snack on appetizers, veggie trays, and lots of homemade treats—including Berlinerkranser (Berlin wreath) cookies, from the Johnsons' Norwegian heritage—while we work together to set the table and make dinner. Before we eat, we all sit down (at two *long* tables) and sing a simple family tradition song, "Father, We Thank Thee." It is absolutely beautiful.

On the menu is roast turkey, mashed potatoes (with soooo much butter—my fave), gravy, green bean casserole, and Norwegian potato bread, which is called lefse. I'm not much of a dessert person (unless it's doughnuts or something *really* amazing), so I usually fill up on all the savory things during the holidays, like my other glorious favorite appetizer . . . spinach dip and sourdough bread. But Amma's homemade apple pie is out of this world, so I need at least one bite.

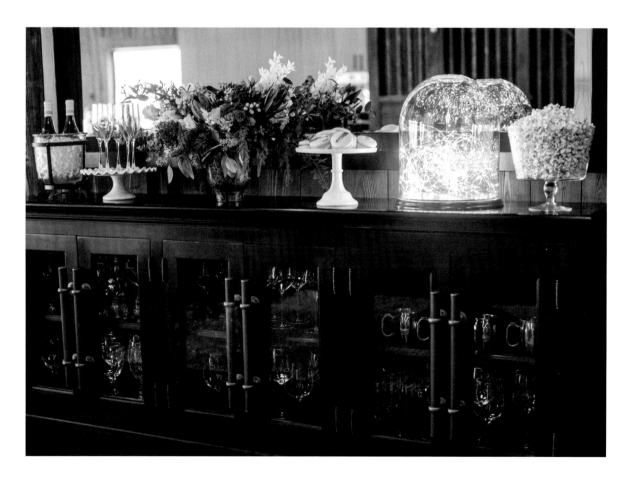

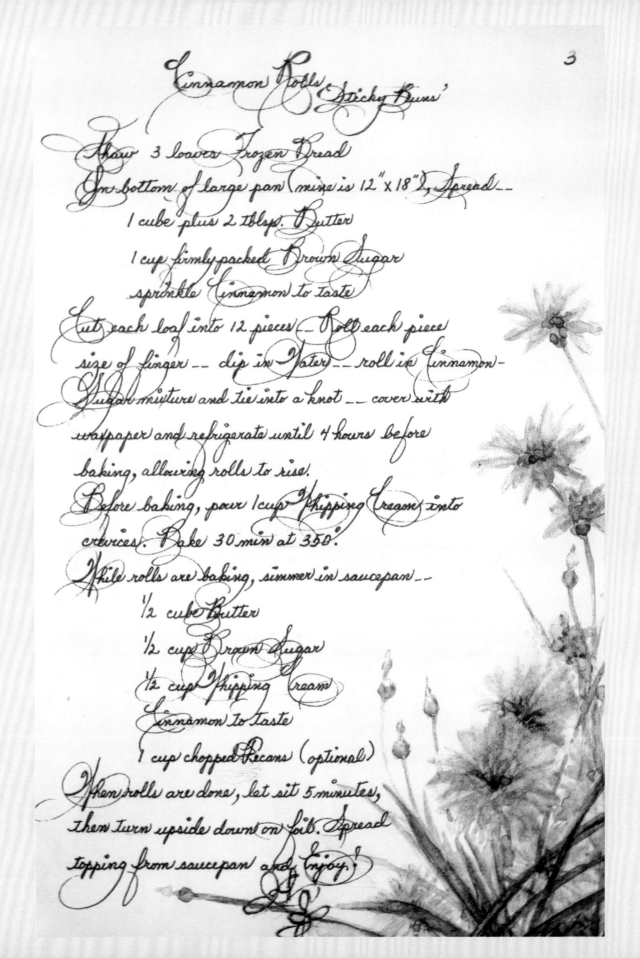

Cinnamon Rolls 'Sticky Buns'

Thaw 3 loaves Frozen Bread

In bottom of large pan (mine is 12" X 18"), Spread __

    1 cube plus 2 tblsp. Butter

    1 cup firmly packed Brown Sugar

    sprinkle Cinnamon to taste

Cut each loaf into 12 pieces __ Roll each piece size of finger __ dip in Water __ roll in Cinnamon-Sugar mixture and tie into a knot __ cover with waxpaper and refrigerate until 4 hours before baking, allowing rolls to rise.

Before baking, pour 1 cup Whipping Cream into crevices. Bake 30 min at 350°.

While rolls are baking, simmer in saucepan __

    ½ cube Butter

    ½ cup Brown Sugar

    ½ cup Whipping Cream

    Cinnamon to taste

    1 cup chopped Pecans (optional)

When rolls are done, let sit 5 minutes, then Turn upside down on foil. Spread topping from saucepan and Enjoy!

For my side of the family, we start with our family's tradition of Christmas breakfast: biscuits and chocolate pudding, or, as my granny calls it, "chocolate gravy" . . . it's divine. When I became best friends with Heather, we were talking about our family holidays and we discovered that (with our families coming from the South), *both* of our families made chocolate gravy for Christmas! I hadn't heard of anyone else making that before. So fun.

Growing up, we made the traditional holiday food for dinner, but my granny loved trying new recipes too. There was always something new to eat, which I loved, as well as my mom's usual chocolate pie.

At our house, Brian and I and the kids have a Christmas tradition of chocolate croissants for breakfast and taking turns reading, telling, or acting out the story of Jesus' birth before we open presents.

With holidays or anything else you celebrate (people, food, health, freedom, season changes, community), make sure your celebration comes from a place of deep gratitude to God. The age-old cheesy phrase "Jesus is the reason for the season" still rings true.

CELEBRATING SOMEONE (OR SOMETHING) SPECIAL

From album release parties to engagement parties to birthday celebrations—it's all about extravagant charcuterie boards for me. I usually do my charcuterie boards with prosciutto, salami, mixed olives (Castelvetrano are my faves!), mixed nuts, dried fruit, Dijon mustard, fig jam, a variety of cheeses (cheddar, blue, Brie, goat, truffle, etc.), Marcona almonds, pickles, and rosemary crackers. Add some sparkly drinks and a dessert board with a variety of chocolates and cookies—and you've got a great party!

Opposite: Grandma Johnson's cinnamon roll recipe

For the dessert boards: I break my favorite dark, milk, and white chocolate bars into 2-inch pieces on one side of the board. Then I add chocolate truffles, a variety of nuts, small cookies, macarons, and fresh berries on the other half of the board.

Throwing a party to celebrate someone or something important is a beautiful way to love your community. Sometimes life can be so full that we don't stop to mark special moments like this, but making time and creating a beautiful space gives the person or the event due honor.

WORSHIP COMMUNITY NIGHTS

We get asked a lot about how we host these nights, but it's pretty simple. We have a budget from the church that includes food for our team for a monthly gathering. So, for worship community night, we invite our entire worship and production team (spouses included) over to our house once a month. I plan the menu with our admin team. (I used to cook the food myself, but now they handle it. So nice!) We start at 6:30 p.m. and spend the first hour just eating and hanging out with everyone. People eating great food, loving one another, and having fun in a beautiful space!

Then we gather together (inside or outside, weather depending), and we pick a couple of our worship leaders and musicians to lead us in an acoustic worship set for thirty to forty-five minutes. After worship, we usually have testimony and prayer request time. Next, we have someone (usually a team member or one of the leaders at church) speak and pray. After that we talk about any news, updates, or business (like introducing new people to the team or praying over anyone who's moving away), and then we let everybody hang out as long as they want. It's the absolute best.

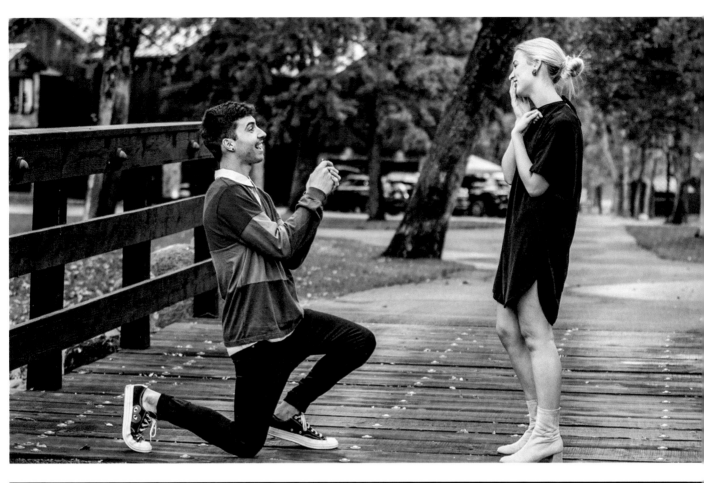

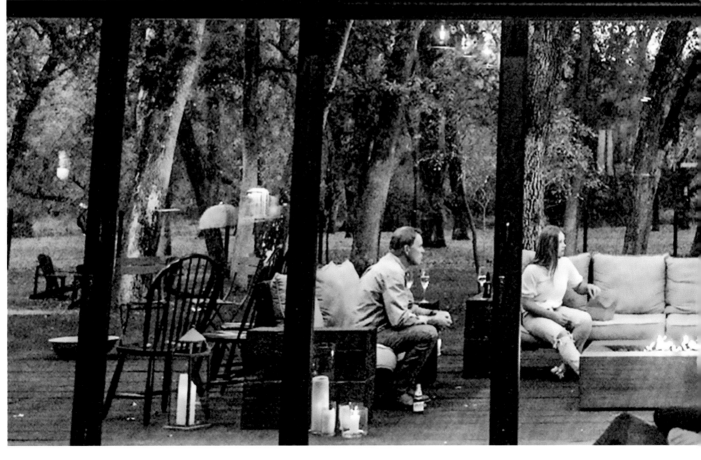

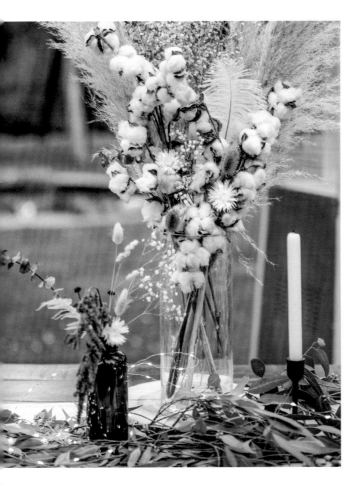
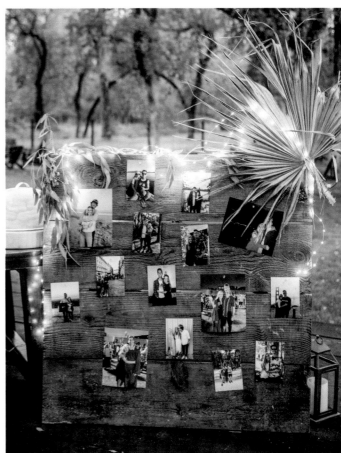
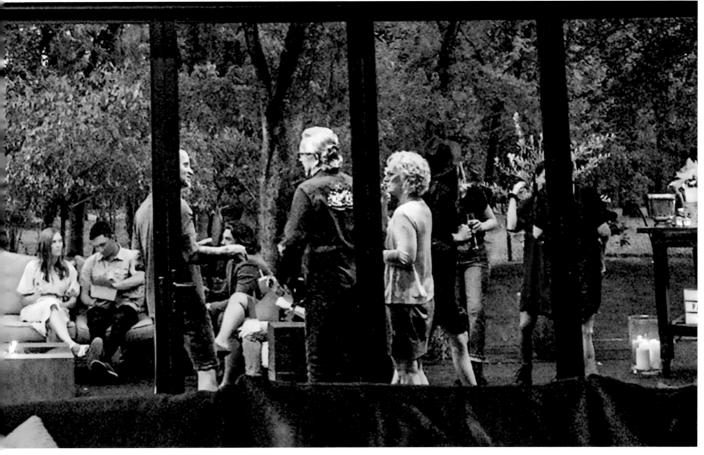

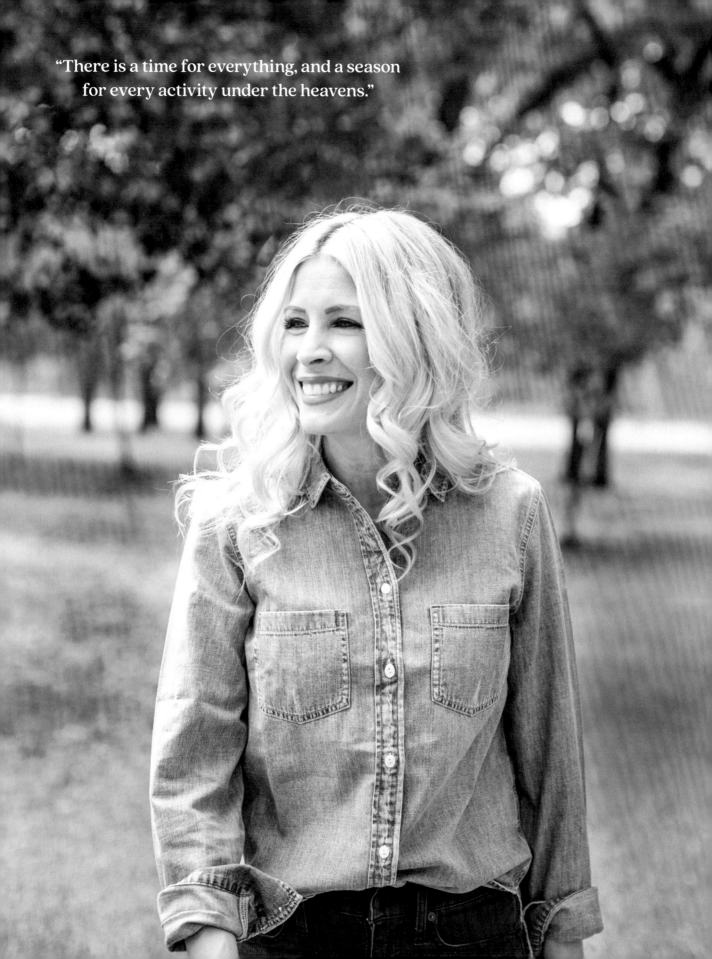

"There is a time for everything, and a season for every activity under the heavens."

Conclusion
ALL THINGS LOVELY

From inspiration and encouragement to some things that may need order in your life, I pray that you've heard God speaking to you and highlighting things He has in store for you as you've read this book.

From getting your house in order, to renovating your heart, to taking the next step in your health journey and reimagining hospitality, I hope this book will help you to bring all things lovely into your life.

Like my dream garden I want to have one day, I will always have a big list of dreams and things I want to accomplish, but I have accepted that I can't do them all at once. Life is like juggling, and we need the Holy Spirit to lead our every moment. When we bring our questions to Him: "Is this something to keep doing?"; "Is this a dream for now or later?"; "Is this healthy or something I need to let go of?" . . . He will answer us. And just like Ecclesiastes 3:1 says, "There is a time for everything, and a season for every activity under the heavens."

God has the perfect timing for everything He's called you to do. *No striving needed.*

Ask God to help you be present and to enjoy where you're at. Don't try to make something happen out of season . . . before it should. Process is important. It's like picking fruit before it's ripe. Or like when you decide to put your Christmas tree up: That's between you and Jesus. Just make sure you're not rushing a season because you're not happy with where you are *right now.*

As we work to put our houses in order, empty our junk drawers, and find emotional, spiritual, and physical health, we need to know that we can't do it alone. My friend Andrew gave me the best advice ever after I had Haley and I was trying to do "all the things." He said, "**Do yourself what only you can do.** Be Brian's wife, the mom of your children, and the leader/songwriter you are . . . **Get help with everything else.** Anyone can get your groceries or clean your house, and you'll bless them by paying them. Take that time and invest it in writing or pastoring or go on a date or play with your kids." I hired a house cleaner that day for a couple of hours a week. It wasn't much, but it was a start, and cutting our fun budget to make that work was worth every penny.

Every year since then, I have worked more and been able to hire more help. So now, yes, I work more, but Instacart delivers our groceries, housekeepers clean . . . and there are Amazon deliveries often. My kids pack their lunches. Friends and family help with our babies so that Brian and I can go on date nights and trips . . . This is the only way I can do "all the things," and there's more time for what I love most: spending time with people I love and helping others through ministry.

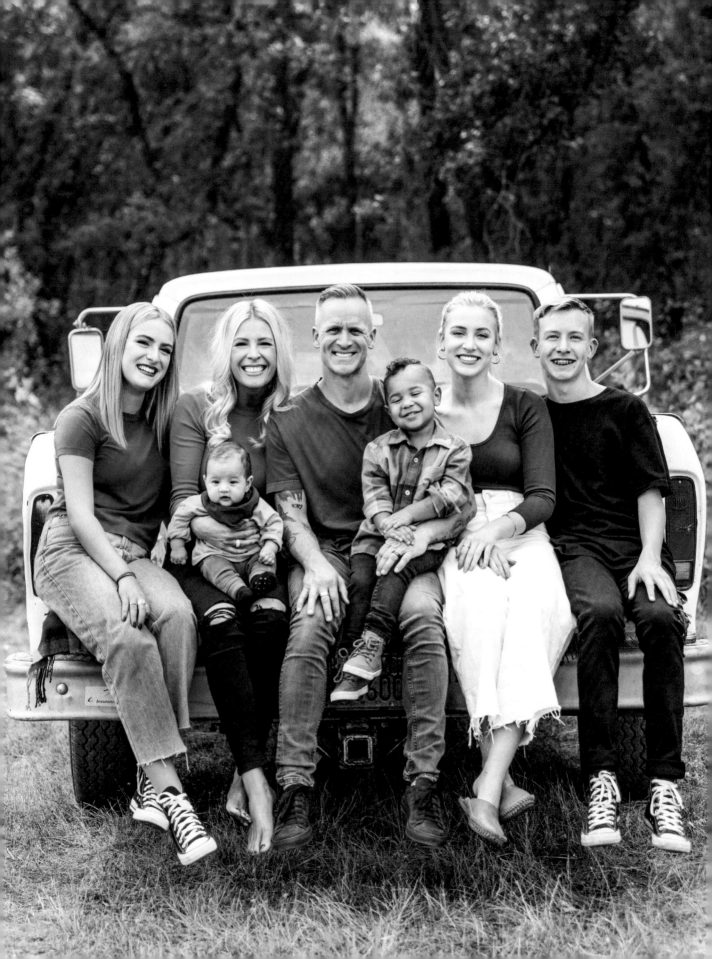

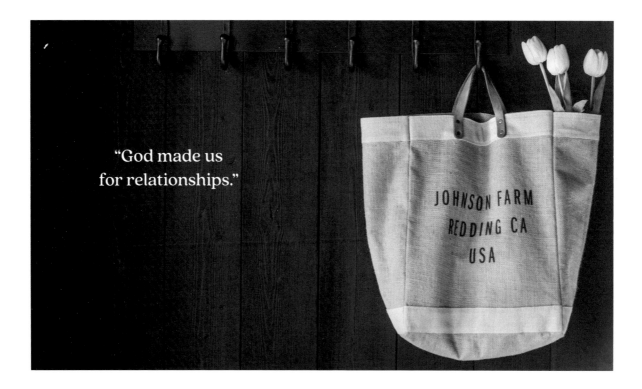

"God made us
for relationships."

No matter what season you're in, invite people into your home, your heart, your life, your mess. God made us for relationships. Our relationship with Him, His Word, and the people He brings into our lives will help us cut anything that isn't lovely, good, or true out of our lives.

> **He cuts off every branch in me that bears no fruit, while every branch that does bear fruit he prunes so that it will be even more fruitful.**
>
> *John 15:2*

Cutting and pruning as applied to our lives never feels good . . . but it IS good . . . and it's vital to our growth and health.

Don't wait until you have *everything* in order to invite people in . . . you never will . . . no one does! Yes, work toward order, but wholeheartedly pursue God and dive into community just as you are.

I hope you hear my heart and my real life in these pages and it inspires you.

I want you to see the place my family lives every day, faded pool toys and all.

I told you stories just like I'd tell my close friends, no filter or holding back.

I don't pretend to be an expert, I just want to help people.

I love order and peace, but I still have chaotic drawers and days sometimes.

I burn food. (I did while shooting the Bolognese for this book. Yes, I did!)

I still say ridiculous things and have to apologize.

I get counseling.

I'm working on reading my Bible more.

I'm working on patience.

I'm working on resting.

I'm working on getting healthier.

I'm working on resting more.

I did another inner healing session last week.

I'm on a journey, just like you, to be healthier emotionally, physically, and spiritually.

There's a lot of nonsense and negativity in the world, but remember, it's all about what you magnify. God's goodness is tangible and everywhere. Magnify it. Magnify Him. And like the verse that this book is anchored on says,

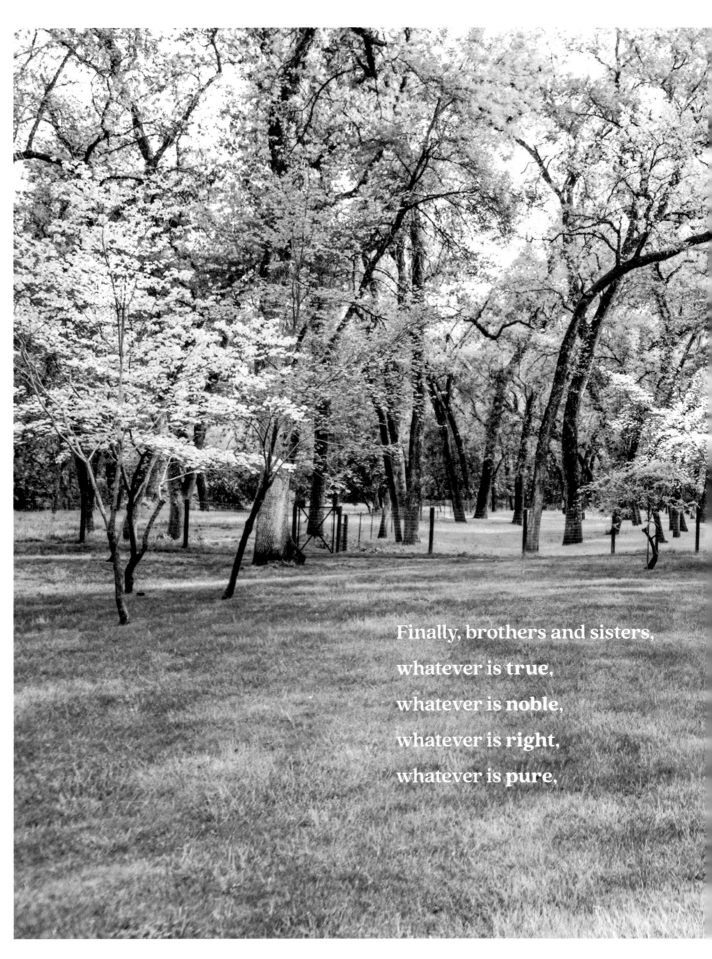

Finally, brothers and sisters,

whatever is **true**,

whatever is **noble**,

whatever is **right**,

whatever is **pure**,

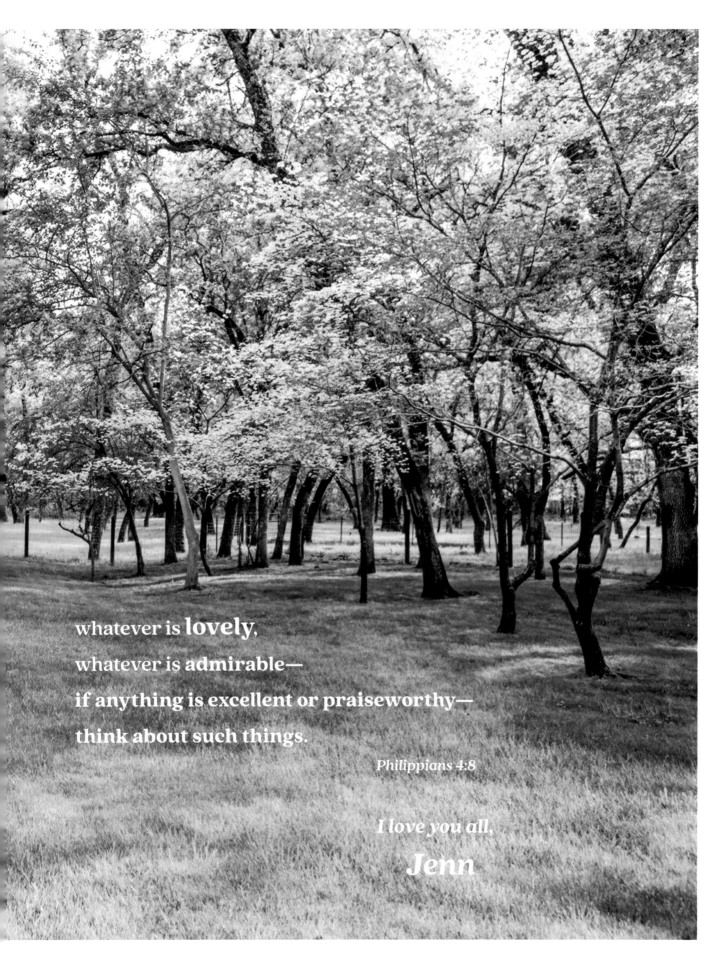

whatever is **lovely**,

whatever is **admirable**—

if anything is excellent or praiseworthy—

think about such things.

Philippians 4:8

I love you all,

Jenn

Acknowledgments

Thank you to everyone who helped me with this
book: Whitney, Esther, Tori, Karen, Morgan,
Danielle, and the rest of the team at Hachette.
I couldn't have done it without you.

And to Heather Armstrong, my best friend, who
took the majority of the photos in this book…you're
amazing, babe! Thank you for your endless hours
of shooting and editing. Lastly, to my incredible
husband for juggling the kids while Heather and I
wrote this book during quarantine.

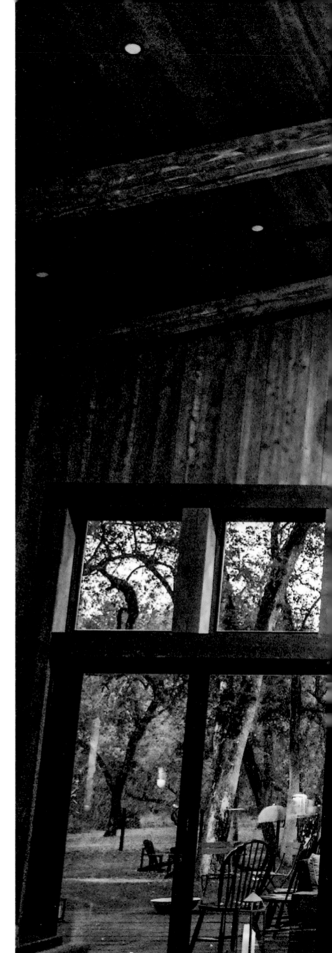

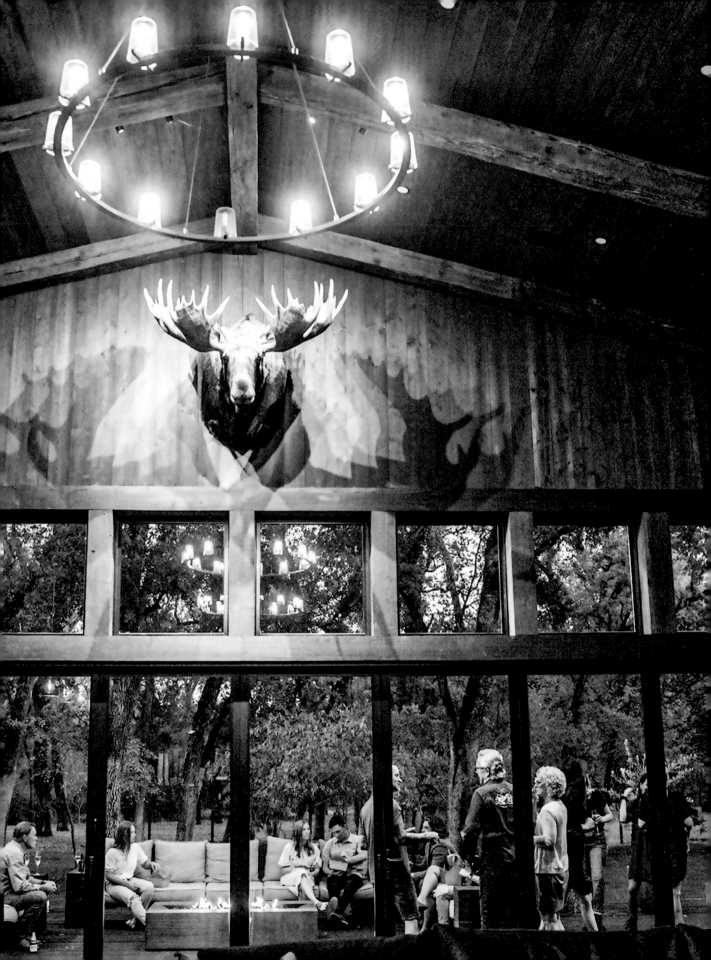

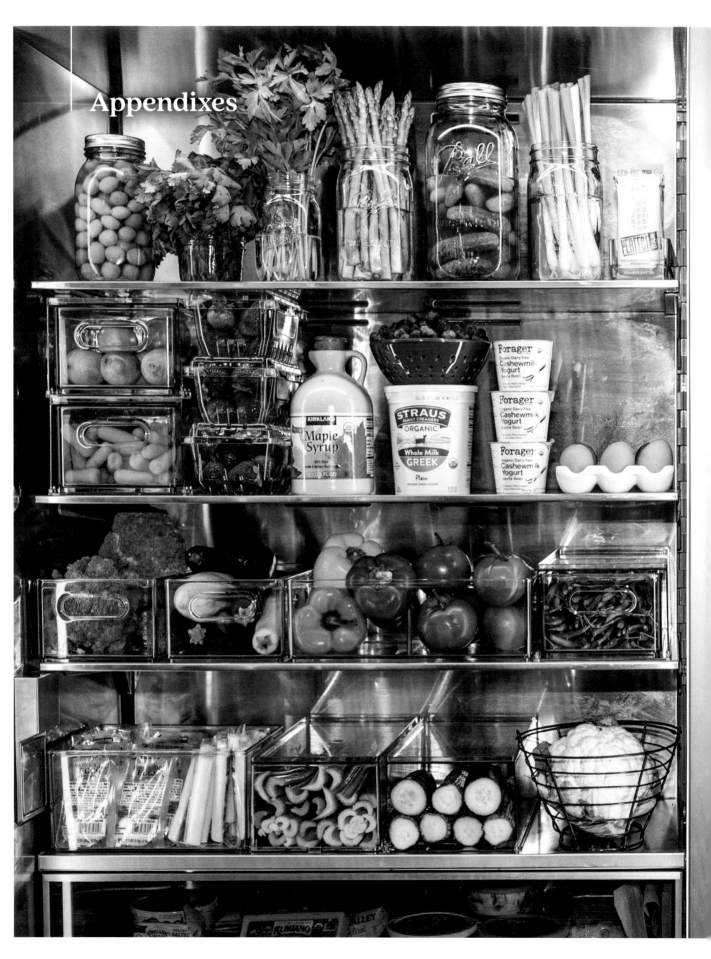

Appendixes

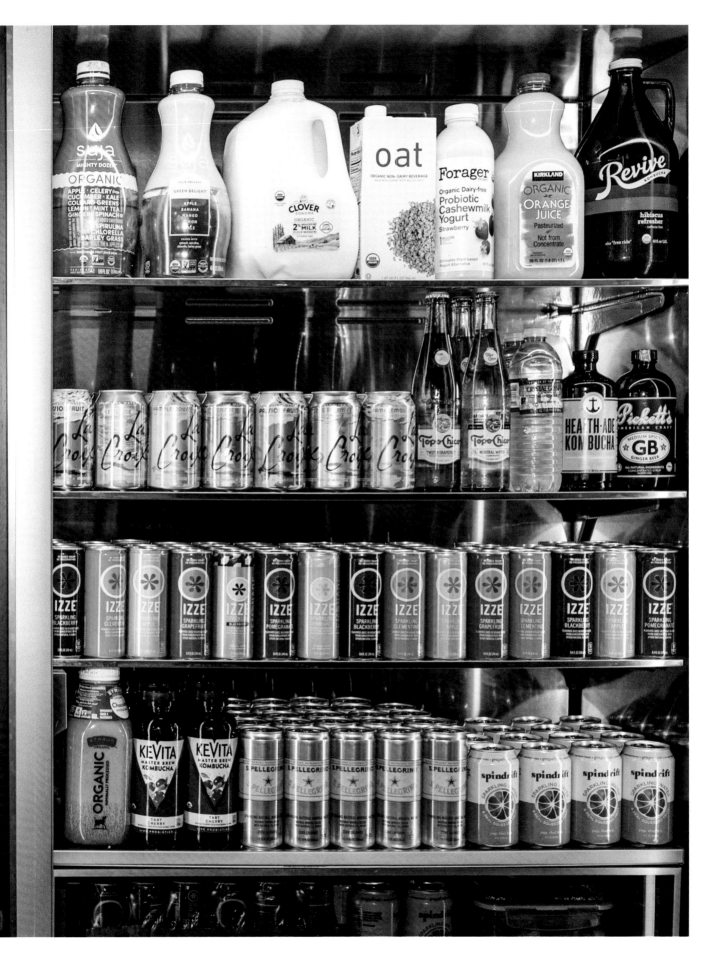

WHAT'S IN MY KITCHEN

Here is a list of healthy items that I try to maintain a supply of in my home.

In the Refrigerator

LIQUIDS:
Sparkling water, sparkling juice, coconut water, Suja juice (green delight, mighty dozen, and uber greens), orange juice, pineapple juice, kombucha, whole milk, coconut milk, oat milk, oat milk creamer, almond milk, maple syrup

CONDIMENTS AND HOT SAUCES:
Barbecue sauce, sriracha, Tapatio, truffle hot sauce, Nandos sauce, Crystal hot sauce, tabasco, chili-garlic sauce, fish sauce, tamarind, Worcestershire, soy sauce, mustard (honey, Dijon, and yellow), basil pesto, Vegenaise, mayonnaise, sweet relish, garlic dill sauerkraut, salsa (red and verde)

PICKLED VEGETABLES:
Pepperoncini, banana pepper rings, Castelvetrano olives, tamed sliced jalapeños, dill pickles, bread and butter pickles, artichoke hearts

DRESSINGS AND BOUILLONS:
Ranch, avocado ranch, blue cheese, caesar, and vinaigrette dressings; chicken, vegetable, and beef bouillons

FRUIT SPREADS:
Strawberry, apricot, fig, blackberry

NUT BUTTERS:
Peanut butter, almond butter, pecan butter, Nuttzo butter

PROTEIN AND DAIRY:
Perfect bars, tahini, cashew milk vanilla yogurt, whole-milk yogurts, eggs, Just Egg substitute, salted butter, unsalted butter, vegan butter, cheddar cheese, mozzarella cheese, vegan mozzarella cheese, American cheese slices, Parmesan, cottage cheese, Mama Chia squeezes

FRUITS:
Apples, mangoes (sliced), applesauce, dried figs, blackberries, raspberries, strawberries, dates

VEGETABLES:
Hummus, green leaf lettuce, romaine lettuce, mushrooms, arugula, spinach, sprouts, broccoli, ginger (minced), garlic (minced and whole cloves), green onions

CARBOHYDRATES:
Gluten-free bread, corn tortillas, flour tortillas, garden wrap tortillas

In the Freezer

VEGETABLES:
Garlic, corn, bell peppers, peas, broccoli, edamame

NUTS:
Cashews, almonds, peanuts, pistachios, pecans, pine nuts

FRUIT:
Strawberries, blueberries, pineapple, mango, bananas, peaches

MEAT, FISH, AND MEAT SUBSTITUTES:
Pork sausage, chicken breasts, whole chickens, ground beef, veggie burgers, quinoa burgers, meatballs, salmon with pesto butter, wild salmon, Atlantic cod, frozen shrimp

MEALS, CARBOHYDRATES, AND SNACKS:

Pizza dough, loaves of bread, cans of biscuits, cauliflower gnocchi, spelt and red quinoa, french fries, steak fries, margherita pizza, mushroom pizza, cheese enchiladas, tamale verde, broccoli/cheddar bowls, lasagna, enchiladas with rice and beans, southwest bowl, chicken flautas, mushroom tortellini, chicken and veggie potstickers, bean and cheese burritos, cilantro lime burritos

DESSERTS:

Vanilla ice cream, chocolate ice cream, raspberry sorbetto, strawberry and mango fruit pops, puff pastries, blueberry waffles

In the Pantry

SNACKS:

Tortilla chips, gluten-free crackers, Nut Thin crackers, pita chips, protein bars, almond berry bites, Lara bars, raisins, cheddar puffs, truffle popcorn, applesauce squeeze packs, cheddar bunnies, fruit strips, veggie straws, Hippea puffs, sunflower seeds, potato chips, dried apricots, seaweed rice cakes, salted popcorn

GRAINS, BEANS, AND PASTA:

Sticky rice, quinoa and brown rice, Basmati rice, white cheddar mac 'n' cheese, lentils, refried beans, black beans, garbanzo beans, rice noodles, ramen noodles, lentils, quinoa

CANNED AND JARRED FRUITS AND VEGETABLES:

Diced tomatoes, peeled tomatoes, pumpkin, jackfruit, blackberry jam, sliced peaches, mandarins, black olives, pineapple chunks, capers, green beans, artichoke hearts, white mushrooms, water chestnuts

ASSORTED CANNED PRODUCTS:

Tomato and garlic sauce, coconut milk, canned chicken, red curry paste, chili, chicken noodle soup, red enchilada sauce, pizza sauce

In the Kitchen Cupboards

BAKING SUPPLIES:

Brown sugar, coconut sugar, flour, whole wheat flour, gluten-free flour, milk powder, baking soda, baking powder, salt, cream of tartar, cornmeal, tapioca powder, arrowroot powder, nutritional yeast

BREAKFAST SUPPLIES:

Oatmeal, Cream of Wheat, grits, granola, chia seeds, dried cranberries, raisins, dried apricots

In a Kitchen Drawer

Potatoes, onions, sweet potatoes

On the Counter

Bananas, avocados

MEASUREMENT EQUIVALENTS

Liquid Measures

1 cup = ½ pint = 8 fluid ounces = 236.5 milliliters

2 cups = 1 pint = 16 fluid ounces = 473 milliliters

4 cups = 1 quart = 32 fluid ounces = 946 milliliters

2 pints = 1 quart = 32 fluid ounces = .946 liter

4 quarts = 1 gallon = 128 fluid ounces = 3.784 liters

Dry Measures

3 teaspoons = 1 tablespoon = ½ ounce = 14.2 grams

2 tablespoons = ⅛ cup = 1 ounce = 28.35 grams

4 tablespoons = ¼ cup = 2 ounces = 56.7 grams

5⅓ tablespoons = ⅓ cup = 2⅔ ounces = 75.6 grams

8 tablespoons = ½ cup = 4 ounces = 113.4 grams

12 tablespoons = ¾ cup = 6 ounces = 170 grams

16 tablespoons = 1 cup = 8 ounces = 226.8 grams

32 tablespoons = 2 cups = 16 ounces = 453.6 grams

64 tablespoons = 4 cups = 32 ounces = 2 pounds = 907 grams

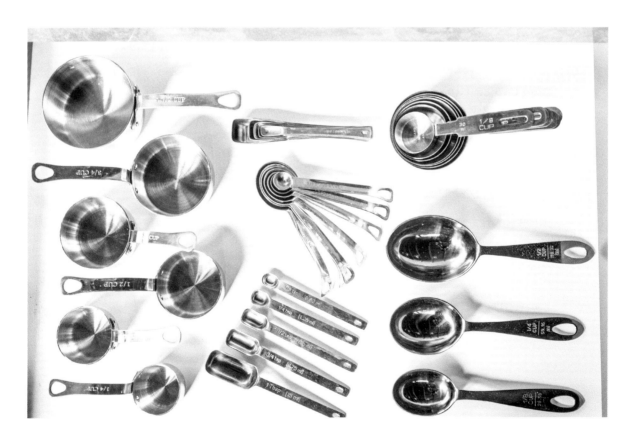

FOOD STORAGE GUIDE

IN THE REFRIGERATOR: Apples, apricots, beets, corn, eggs, grapefruit, kiwi, leeks, lemons, limes, mandarins, mangoes, nectarines, oranges, papayas, passionfruit, peaches, pears, persimmons, plums, pomegranates, quinces, turnips, watermelon, zucchini

IN A SEALED CONTAINER OR BAG, IN THE REFRIGERATOR: Artichokes, arugula, cabbage, cauliflower (keep outer leaves attached), celery, cherries, cilantro, figs (in a sealed container), grapes, green beans, peas, radishes, rhubarb, rosemary, Swiss chard

IN A SEALED CONTAINER LINED WITH A DRY PAPER TOWEL, IN THE REFRIGERATOR: Berries, coffee

WRAPPED IN A DAMP PAPER TOWEL IN A SEALED CONTAINER, IN THE REFRIGERATOR: Kale, kohlrabi, lettuce, mint, spinach, tarragon, thyme (fresh)

IN A PAPER BAG, IN THE REFRIGERATOR: Bell peppers, broccoli, chiles, mushrooms, parsnips

UPRIGHT IN A GLASS OF WATER, IN THE REFRIGERATOR: Asparagus, basil (fresh), green onions, parsley (fresh), watercress

IN THE REFRIGERATOR CRISPER: Carrots (for baby carrots, keep in glass of fresh water to hold color); cucumbers (in a sealed container)

AWAY FROM DIRECT SUNLIGHT UNTIL RIPE; ONCE RIPE, KEEP IN THE REFRIGERATOR: Avocados, bananas, tomatoes

IN THE FREEZER: Flour, garlic, ginger (unpeeled), nuts (in a sealed container or bag), rice

IN A COOL, DARK, DRY PLACE: Eggplants, onions, potatoes, pumpkins, squash (acorn/butternut/spaghetti), sweet potatoes, yams

Helpful Food Storage Facts

FIG FACTS: While figs are best eaten the same day they are picked, if slightly unripe, they can be stored on a plate lined with fig leaves.

GREEN ONIONS FOR YOUR GARDEN: If the tiny white roots of your green onions begin to grow, you can plant the stalks in your garden and then you'll have fresh green onions for a year or two! Just trim the green as needed.

QUICK-RIPENING YOUR AVOCADOS: Put them in a container with an apple, pear, nectarine, kiwi, apricot, plum, or peach! These fruits produce a gas called ethylene that accelerates the avocado ripening.

USING CRISPER DRAWERS: Most refrigerators have these, and you can adjust the humidity for individual drawers. Generally, low humidity is best for fruit, and high humidity is best for vegetables.

A GOOD FRIDGE TEMP: An internal temperature around 35°F is best for optimal freshness.

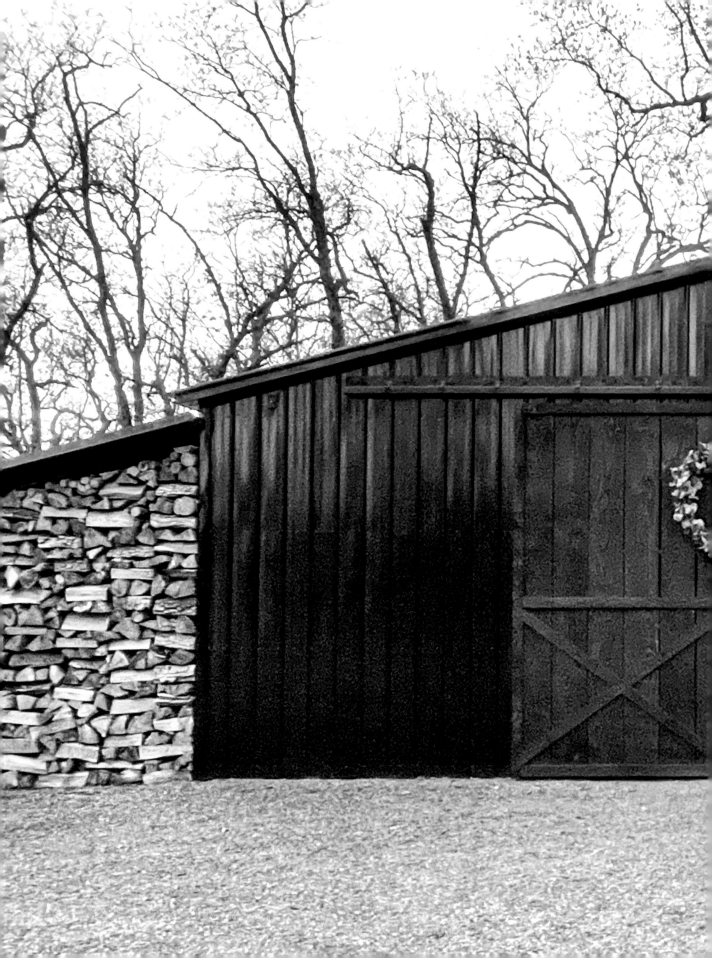

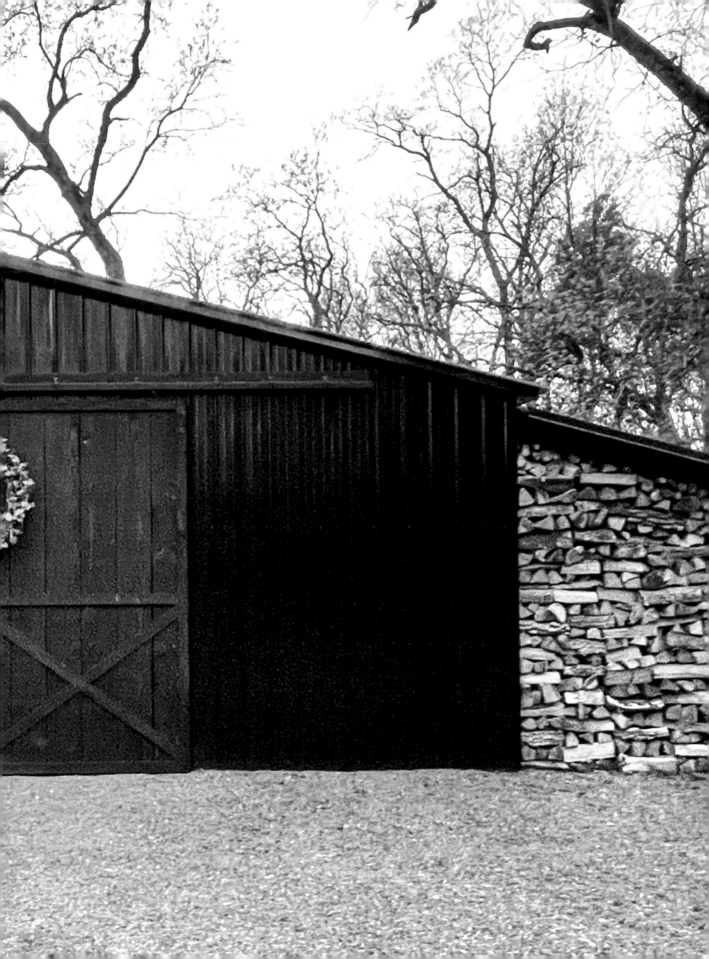

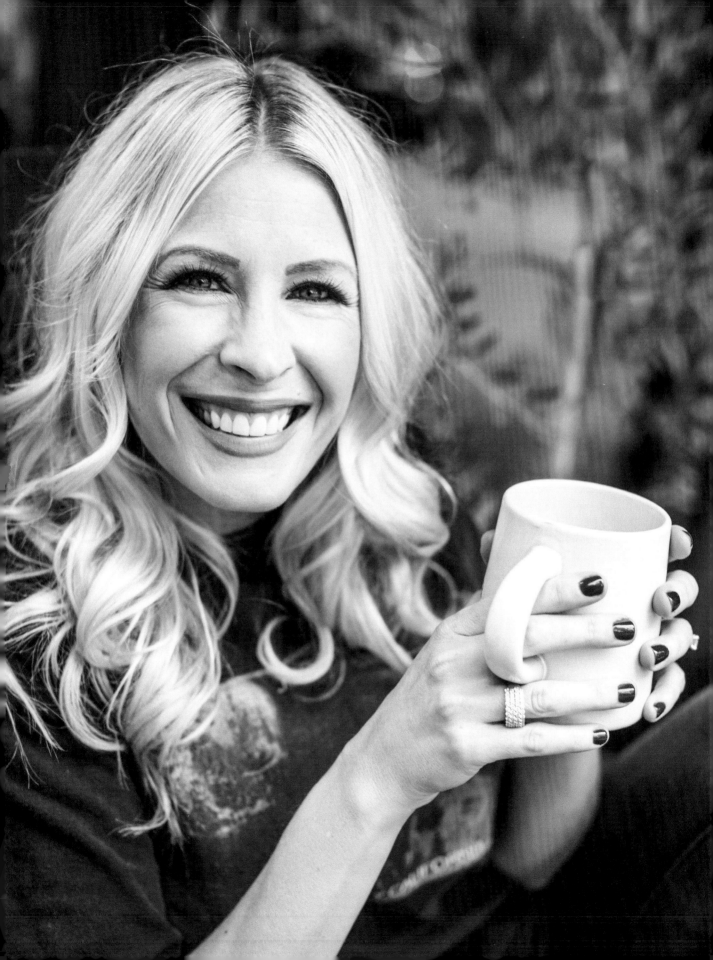

About the Author

Jenn Johnson is the cofounder of Bethel Music and WorshipU along with her husband, Brian Johnson. She has been involved in the production of more than fifteen albums that have influenced the culture of worship across the global church. Jenn is the founder of "Lovely by Jenn Johnson," a lifestyle brand intended to inspire, equip, and engage women of all ages to thrive. The Johnsons also head Bethel Church Worship Ministry and are committed to cultivating community and fostering unity among worship leaders from around the world. Jenn is passionate about living a lifestyle of worship built on vulnerability, purity, and connection to community and leadership. Brian and Jenn live in Redding, California, with their five amazing kids, Haley, Téa, Braden, Ryder Moses, and Malachi Judah. Jenn continues to speak and lead worship at home and around the world.

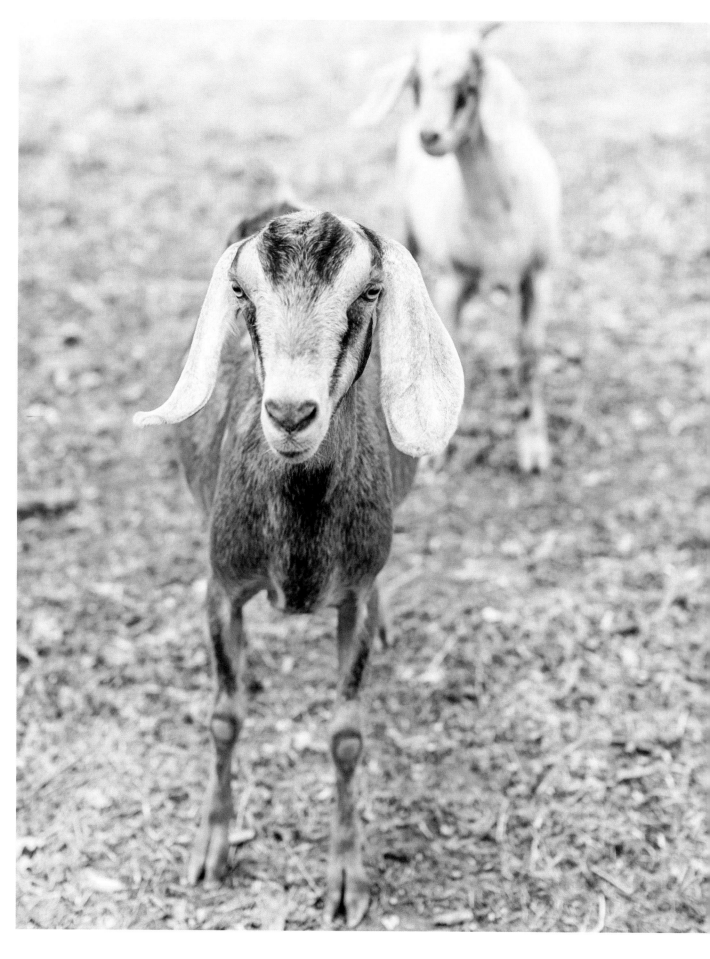